Back & Neck Pain Relief

Dr. David M. Warwick

Doctor of Chiropractic

Printed in the United States of America
First Printing: December 2015
Reprint June 2017

Short Term Care
for Your Back & Neck Pain...

And Not One Single Visit More

For More Information Visit:
www.DrDavidWarwick.com

Table of Contents

Introduction

If you have been suffering with back or neck pain or even both you are probably confused about what to do next. You are probably asking yourself questions like the following:

"What is wrong with my back or neck?"

"I've tried 'xyz' treatment and it didn't work?

"Who can I go to that I trust?"

"How much will it cost?"

"Will my insurance cover, and if not, how much will I pay?"

"How long will it take?"

If you or someone you care about has any of these concerns, please keep reading this special Back & Neck Pain Book.

Hi. My name is David M. Warwick, D.C., and I've been helping people with Back and Neck Pain and even headaches get fast and effective relief from back & neck pain, the stresses of daily living, injuries or even sometimes the, "I Don't Know Syndromes" for almost 20 years.

Back and neck pain is 'very real" problem affecting almost 80% of you including me at some point in our lives and costs our communities billions in health care, disability and loss of work dollars.

Maybe your doctor told you 'take this and give it a couple of weeks' ... 'you'll be fine' ... or maybe you even got 'the look'.

Well it's not fine. You are not fine. You hurt. And you want to feel better and go about your life.

Maybe your back or neck hurt when you work at the computer, when the dog pulls hard on the leash, when you have the 'honey-do-list' around the house or yard...maybe sleep has become more difficult with a lot of tossing and turning and not be able to get comfortable or even worse just the act of showering or getting dressed has become a 'a careful circus act'. Even more so now there are headaches growing worse or it's been going on for years on months or weeks.

Maybe you noticed how your back or neck moves differently and it's getting worse. Maybe you know what caused it or don't.

Does this sound familiar?

Well, you have had enough. You want to take action and get help. Now!

It's quite surprising when you look at back and neck pain researches how it impacts the entire body. You probably didn't think that headaches, carpal tunnel syndrome, fibromyalgia or even whiplash injury are part of that pain, but they are...

Over the past almost 20 years I have treated hundreds of patients with whiplash injuries, and I believe the systematic approach we use in my office to be very effective at helping patients Feel Better Faster.

Don't take my word for it.....I have included a sample of my many satisfied patients that have written testimonials. I have also included a collection of the most relevant articles I have published in my popular "In Good Hands" newsletter over the last few years.

It's easy to make your first appointment with me. All you have to do is call my office today at **(360) 951-4504** and schedule an evaluation to see if we can help you. We'll do everything possible to get you in the same day...even if we have to stay late or work through lunch! You're too young to suffer with back and neck pain. Let's handle that today. Ok, here's what to do right now...

Call (360) 951-4504 Today!

My staff and I would love to work with you. All you have to do is call my office right now and we will schedule a time that's convenient for you! I have the friendliest staff you will ever meet and we are all specially trained in handling the often-confusing paperwork and forms that need to be filled out.

We look forward to helping you Feel Better Faster.

David M. Warwick, D.C.

P.S. To the best of my ability, I agree to provide my patients convenient, affordable, and mainstream Chiropractic care. I will not use unnecessary long-term treatment plans and/or therapies. – Dr. David Warwick, D.C.

This book has been carefully prepared to educate those who have suffered back and neck pain and even headaches involving the spine. The information presented is for general health education only. Individual health concerns should be addressed with a knowledgeable and licensed health care provider.

Why Does My Back Hurt?

It's been said that if you haven't had back pain, just wait, because (statistically) someday you will! The following list is a list of "causes" that can be easily "fixed" to reduce your risk for a back pain episode.

1. MATTRESS: Which type of mattress is best? The "short answer": there is no single mattress (style or type) for all people, primarily due to body type, size, gender, and what "feels good." TRY laying on a variety of mattresses (for several minutes on your back and sides) and check out the difference between coiled, inner springs, foam (of different densities), air, waterbeds, etc. The thickness of a mattress can vary from 7 to 18 inches (~17-45 cm) deep. Avoid mattresses that feel like you're sleeping in a hammock! A "good" mattress should maintain your natural spinal curves when lying on your sides or back (avoid stomach sleeping in most cases). Try placing a pillow between the knees and "hug" a pillow when side sleeping, as it can act like a "kick stand" and prevent you from rolling onto your stomach. If your budget is tight, you can "cheat" by placing a piece of plywood between the mattress and box spring as a short-term fix.

2. SHOES: Look at the bottom of your favorite pair of shoes and check out the "wear pattern." If you have worn out soles or heels, you are way overdue for a new pair or a "re-sole" by your local shoe cobbler! If you work on your feet, then it's even more important for both managing and preventing LBP!

3. DIET: A poor diet leads to obesity, which is a MAJOR cause of LBP. Consider the Paleo or Mediterranean Diet and STAY AWAY from fast food! Identify the two or three "food abuses" you have embraced and eliminate them – things with empty calories like soda, ice cream, chips... you get the picture! Keeping your BMI (Body Mass Index) between 20 and 25 is the goal! Positive "side-effects" include increased longevity, better overall health, and an improved quality of life!

4. EXERCISE: The most effective self-help approach to LBP management is exercise. Studies show those who exercise regularly hurt less, see doctors less, have a higher quality of life, and just feel better! This dovetails with diet in keeping your weight in check as well. Think of hamstring stretches and core strengthening as important LBP managers – USE PROPER TECHNIQUE AND FORM; YOUR DOCTOR OF CHIROPRACTIC CAN GUIDE YOU IN THIS PROCESS!

5. POSTURE: Another important "self-help" trick of the trade is to avoid sitting slumped over with an extreme forward head carriage positions. Remember that every inch your head pokes forwards places an additional ten pounds (~4.5 kg) of load on your upper back muscles to keep your head upright, and sitting slumped increases the load on your entire back!

Is Sitting BAD for My Back?

A major manufacturer of workstations reports that 86% of work computer users have to sit all day, and when they do rise from sitting, more than half (56%) use food as the excuse to get up and move. In addition to sitting at work, for meals, and commuting to/from work, 36% sit another one to two hours watching TV, 10% sit one to two hours for gaming, 25% sit one to two hours for reading/lounging, and 29% use their home computer for one to two hours. In summary, the average American sits for thirteen hours a day and sleep for eight hours. That's a total of 21 hours a day off their feet!

The manufacturer's survey also notes 93% of work computer users don't know what "Sitting Disease" is but 74% believe that sitting too much can lead to an early death. "Sitting Disease" represents the ill-effects of an overly sedentary lifestyle and includes conditions like "metabolic syndrome" (obesity and diabetes), which is rapidly becoming more prevalent, especially in the young – even in adolescence and teenagers! Recently, the American Medical Association (AMA) adopted a policy encouraging employers, employees, and others to sit less citing the many risks associated with sitting including (but not limited to): diabetes, cancer, obesity, and cardiovascular disease. Standing is SO MUCH BETTER as it burns more calories than sitting, tones muscles, improves posture, increases blood flow, reduces blood sugar, and improves metabolism. Standing is frequently overlooked as "an exercise" and it's both simple and easy to do!

So, what about the low back and sitting? You guessed it – sitting is hard on the back! The pressure inside of our disks, those "shock absorbers" that lie between each vertebra in our spine (22 disks in total) is higher when we sit compared with simply standing or lying down. It's estimated that when we lay down, the pressure on our disks is the lowest at 25mm. When lying on one side, it increases to 75mm, standing increases disk pressure to 100mm, and bending over from standing pushes disk pressure to 220mm. When we sit with good posture, our disk pressure may reach 140mm but that can increase to 190mm with poor posture. To help relieve the pressure on our disks, experts recommend: 1) Getting up periodically and standing; 2) Sitting back in your chair and avoiding slouched positions; 3) Placing a lumbar roll (about the size of your forearm) behind the low back and chair/car seat; and 4) Changing your position frequently when sitting.

Because certain low back conditions "favor" one position over another, these "rules" may need modification. For example, most herniated disk patients prefer low back extension while bending over or slouching hurts. In those with lumbar sprain/strains, bending forwards usually feels good and extension hurts. Modifying your position to the one that is most comfortable is perhaps the best advice.

What's that Tingling in My Leg?

When you think of low back pain, you may visualize a person half-bent over with their hand on the sore spot of their back. Since many of us have experienced low back pain during our lifetime, we can usually relate to a personal experience and recall how limited we were during the acute phase of our last LBP episode. However, when the symptoms associated with LBP are different, such as tingling or a shooting pain down one leg, it can be both confusing and worrisome – hence the content of this month's article!

Let's look at the anatomy of the low back to better understand where these symptoms originate. In the front of the spine (or the part more inside of the body), we have the big vertebral bodies and shock absorbing disks that support about 80% of our weight. At the back of each vertebra you'll find the spinous and transverse processes that connect to the muscles and ligaments in the back to the spine. Between the vertebral body and these processes are the tiny boney pieces called the pedicles. The length of the pedicle partially determines the size of the holes where the nerves exit the spine.

When the pedicles are short (commonly a genetic cause), the exiting nerves can be compressed due to the narrowed opening. This is called foraminal spinal stenosis. This compression usually occurs later in life when osteoarthritis and/or degenerative disk disease further crowds these "foramen" where the nerves exit the spine. Similarly, short pedicles can narrow the "central canal" where the spinal cord travels up and down the spine from the brain. Later in life, the combined effects of the narrow canal plus disk bulging, osteoarthritic spurs, and/or thickening or calcification of ligaments can add up to "central spinal stenosis." The symptoms associated with spinal stenosis (whether it's foraminal or central) include difficulty walking due to a gradual increase in tingling, heavy, crampy, achy and/or sore feeling in one or both legs. The tingling in the legs associated with spinal stenosis is called "neurogenic claudication" and must be differentiated from "vascular claudication", which feels similar but is caused from lack of blood flow to the leg(s) as opposed to nerve flow.

At a younger age, tingling in the legs can be caused by either a bulging or herniated lumbar disk or it can be referred pain from a joint – usually a facet or sacroiliac joint. The main difference in symptoms between nerves vs. joint leg tingling symptoms is that nerve pinching from a

18

deranged disk is located in a specific area in the leg such as the inside or outside of the foot. In other words, the tingling can be traced fairly specifically in the leg. Tingling from a joint is often described as a deep, "inside the leg," generalized achy-tingling that can affect the whole leg and/or foot or it may stop at the knee, but it's more difficult to describe by the patient as it's less geographic or specific in its location. Chiropractic management of all these conditions offers a non-invasive, effective form of non-surgical, non-drug care and is the recommended in LBP guidelines as an option when treating these conditions.

Why Does My Back Hurt Part 2?

Last time, we discussed common causes of back pain including mattresses, shoes, diet, exercise, and posture. Here are some additional considerations…

6. OFFICE CHAIR: Because of vast differences between people's height, weight, body type, and preference, it's difficult — if not impossible — to find a one-size-fits-all solution when it comes to office chairs! In the ideal world, the option to sit, stand, walk, and stretch as needed would be perfect but this simply is not reality! Low back pain (LBP) from sitting is common due to the excess pressure it places on the joints and disks (the "shock-absorbers" of the spine). Here are some remedies: 1) Find a chair that FITS YOU. 2) Get up and move at least once every hour (set the timer on your smartphone as a reminder). 3) Place the computer monitor directly in front of you and keyboard/mouse so the elbows bend only 90°. 4) Keep your feet on the floor at your desk (use an upside down box if you have short legs). 5) Perform "in the chair" stretches when your timer goes off!

7. BODY TYPE: We've discussed obesity as an obvious cause of back pain, but other factors are important as well. A very common cause of back pain for women is breast size. Here, the topic of a supportive bra is important, as carrying more weight in front of you adds additional stress on the back and shoulders.

8. SHOULDER BAGS: Back pain can be caused and/or perpetuated by a heavy purse, bag, briefcase, and even a thick wallet in the back pocket! To keep your eyes level, your body has to compensate and assume a less-than-ideal posture that may place unnecessary stress on your back! So before leaving the house today, CLEAN OUT that bag and/or put your wallet in a front pocket and lessen the load on your spine!

9. SMOKING: Smoking can reduce the amount of oxygen that reaches your cells, which can cause them to function at a less than optimal state. You've perhaps heard that a conscientious back surgeon will NEVER operate on a smokers' back due to both the prolonged healing time and subsequent bad outcomes. So in addition to giving your heart, lungs, and those around you a break, if you want your lower back to heal, STOP SMOKING! Studies also show smokers are TWICE as likely to develop LBP compared with non-smokers, so quit. Better yet, DON'T START in the first place!

10. STRESS & DEPRESSION: Remember, "Health" is a balance between structure, chemistry, and mental factors. Stress increases muscle tightness and alters posture in a way that can lead to or exacerbate existing LBP. Exercise, meditate, eat smart, and resolve your differences with family members and friends to minimize this problem!

When needed, your doctor of chiropractic can refer you for counseling!

11. ERGONOMICS: How we "fit" into our job, lifting properly, workstation set up, work pace, and work stressors ALL play into LBP management. Have an assessment to see what can be fixed!

A Low Back Pain Warning
You Better Not Ignore…

Low back pain (LBP) typically results from relatively "benign" causes, meaning it's usually safe to wait and try conservative / non-emergency care first. However, there are a handful of times when prompt medical emergency management is appropriate, and it's important that everyone is aware of these uncommon but dangerous and sometimes deadly causes of LBP, hence the purpose of this article.

"Red flags" trace back to the 1980s and 1990s, so this is not a "new" topic. In fact, guidelines for the care of LBP that have been published around the world ALL commonly state the anyone exhibiting these "red flags" needs to be promptly diagnosed and referred for emergent care. The common conditions cited in these guidelines include (but are not limited to): 1) Cancer, 2) Cauda equine syndrome, 3) Infection, 4) Fracture. The patient's history can sometimes uncover suspicion of these four conditions BETTER than a routine physical examination, though a definitive diagnosis is usually made only after special diagnostic tests have been completed including (but not limited to) imaging (x-ray, MRI, CT, PET scans), blood tests, bone scans, and more.

1) Cancer: a) Past history of cancer. b) Unexplained weight loss (>10 kg within 6 months). c) Age over 50 or under age 18. d) Failure to respond to usual care (therapy). e) Pain that persists for four to six weeks. f) Night pain or pain at rest.

2) Infection: a) Persistent fever (>100.4° F). b) Current/recent URI (upper respiratory tract infection like pneumonia) or UTI (urinary tract or kidney infection). b) History of intravenous drug abuse. c) Severe back pain. d) Lumbar spine surgery within the past year. e) Recent bacterial infection (cellulitis or persistent wound – e.g., a decubitus ulcer or "pressure sore" in the low back region). f) Immunocompromised states such as those caused by systemic corticosteroids, organ transplant medications, diabetes mellitus, human immunodeficiency virus (HIV).

3) Cauda Equina Syndrome: a) Urinary incontinence or retention. b) Saddle anesthesia. c) Anal sphincter tone decrease or fecal incontinence. d) Bilateral lower extremity weakness or numbness. e) Progressive neurologic deficit or loss – major muscle weakness or sensory deficit.

4) Fracture: a) Prolonged corticosteroid use. b) Age >70. c) History of Osteoporosis (poor bone density). d) Mild trauma over age 50. e) Major trauma at any age (such as a fall).

Another red flag is an Abdominal Aortic Aneurism. Signs include: a) Abdominal pulsations. b) Hardening of the arteries (atherosclerotic vascular disease). c) Pain at rest or night time pain. d) Age >60.

Back & Neck Pain Relief As Fast As Possible?

Doctors Approach to Back & Neck Pain Gets Rave Reviews

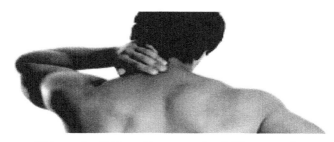

Lacey/Olympia WA – It's amazing! The word spread so fast the phone was ringing off the hook. Back and neck pain sufferers came out of the woodwork.

It's incredible how word of mouth travels like wildfire when a doctor actually gives patients what they want...the way they want it...at a price they can afford.

That's exactly what Dr. David Warwick does. Dr. Warwick is a Chiropractor who practices in Lacey and has a very refreshing philosophy. With that in mind, he tries to get back & neck pain patients out of pain...as fast as possible...with the least amount of treatment for the least amount of expense.

And it is Working...

Dr. Warwick does not believe in long term chiropractic treatment unless absolutely necessary that can cost thousands of dollars. Every patient is accepted in a visit to visit basis without any commitment or obligation what-so-ever.

"The biggest advantage for patients is that they can receive chiropractic treatment care on a visit by visit basis and only continue if they like it and it is working for them"....says Dr. Warwick

With all the problems and uncertainty with healthcare today, this approach has created quite a buzz in Lacey. Back and neck pain sufferers now a have a Doctor of Chiropractic that they can work with and they can afford. But most of all – offers short-term care without any long term commitment.

Here's what Dr. Warwick has to say..."To the best of my ability, I agree to provide my patients convenient, affordable, and mainstream Chiropractic care. I will not use unnecessary long-term treatment plans and/or therapies."

If you suffer with neck and/or back pain and would like a consultation, call **360-951-4504** or **walk in; no appointment needed.** It's no charge and no further obligation to receive care. <u>Contact</u> Dr. David Warwick today!

Why Do I Have Neck or Back Pain?

In a study that looked at stress and how people who seek chiropractic care perceive it, researchers wrote that psychosocial stress, "…pervades modern life and is known to have an impact on health. Pain, especially chronic back pain, is influenced by stress." Here, ten different chiropractic clinics reported results tallied from 138 patients who were given questionnaires about stress and its association with their current condition.

Of interest, more than 30% categorized themselves as being "moderately to severely stressed," and over 50% felt that stress had a moderate or greater effect on their presenting complaint. Further, about 71% of the patients felt that a stress management approach would be useful to help them cope and 44% were interested in taking a "self-development program to enhance their stress management skills."

The study concluded that: 1) patient perceptions are known to be important in management approaches and treatment outcomes; 2) in this study, about 1/3 of patients presenting perceived themselves as being moderately or severely stressed; and 3) interventions that reduce stress or the patient's perception of being stressed may be an important and valid "intervention" in patient management.

So, how do doctors of chiropractic do this? First is pain management, which is often at the core of a current heightened stress level, as it can push the stress level "over the edge." But just managing pain doesn't always work by itself, and doctors of chiropractic will often intervene with nutritional recommendations such as educating the patient about an "anti-inflammatory diet," and the use of vitamin and/or herbal approaches specific to stress management, including specific nutritional approaches to balancing neurotransmitter levels. Other approaches may include the use of various calming techniques that can be employed at times when patients are "stressed" and can be used during the day during these "stressful moments."

There are even "calming apps" to help de-stress and clear the mind available for your smartphone! Just as there are apps to measure your steps, calories, or METS burned during the day, these apps are specific for calming and reducing stress! Here are the names of a few that are FREE for you to investigate and consider (Web, Android, or iOS): MindMeister, Breath2Relax, White Noise Lite, Calm, Diaro, Headspace, Relax, Guided Meditations, and more. Give one of these a try as it is clear we all focus far too little on stress management!

Spinal Manipulation AFTER Surgery HELPS!

Unfortunately, low back pain (LBP) is something MOST of us cannot avoid. There is solid evidence that chiropractic care is one of the most effective methods of treating LBP, but there are times when a referral for surgery is needed. What about manipulative therapy (MT) AFTER surgery? Is this a good idea? Does it help?

In March 2015, an article published in the Journal of Back and Musculoskeletal Rehabilitation discussed the pros and cons of MT after lumbar open laser micro discectomy, a common surgical technique used to treat patients with a pinched nerve due to a herniated lumbar disk. Unfortunately, patients who undergo this procedure can experience early post-surgical physical disability that reduces their ability to perform required daily activities. For this reason, the objective of this study was to look at whether early individualized spinal manipulation would reduce the occurrence of post-surgical disability. To do this, 21 patients (aged 25-69) who had a micro discectomy were randomly placed into either a spinal manipulation or an active control group. Manipulation was performed two to three weeks after surgery, at two times a week for four weeks.

The researchers found patients in the MT group experienced a 55% reduction in disability while those in the control group reported a 5% increase in disability! Also, leg pain was reduced by 55% in the MT group compared with only 9% in the control group. This pilot study concluded that while a larger-scale study is recommended, the findings indicate that manipulation "...may be an important option for post-operative management after spinal surgery."

This is yet another testimony that spinal manipulation can not only help many people avoid surgery, but it can also significantly reduce or eliminate back pain and disability AFTER surgery! Spinal manipulation is the most common treatment approach performed routinely by chiropractors. And although other healthcare professionals are showing an increasingly greater interest in learning this skill, manipulation must be performed on a regular, concentrated basis in order to obtain the best outcomes or therapeutic results for patients. So, regardless if you have or have not had surgery for LBP, the benefits of chiropractic and spinal manipulation are recognized as a recommended course of treatment!

Low Back Pain? Should You Take An NSAID?

Statistics suggest that low back pain (LBP) will plague most of us at some point in our lives, if it hasn't already. Most healthcare professions that manage patients with low back pain focus on pain management. In fact, studies have reported that 67% of patient satisfaction is driven by pain elimination. One of the most common strategies for reducing pain is managing inflammation. The "easiest" way to do this (according to the many TV commercials and magazine advertisements) is to take one of the many non-steroidal anti-inflammatory drugs (NSAIDs) such as Ibuprofen (Advil, Nuprin), Piroxicam Flurbiprofen, and Indomethacin. Let's take a closer look to see if this is a good or bad idea!

In a recent March 2015 article, researchers investigated the use of NSAIDs between 1993 and 2012 in patients who had fractures that failed to heal, technically called "non-union fractures." They found that non-union fractures increased during years when NSAID use was increasingly recommended for patients with fractures and dropped in years when NSAID use declined. This isn't the first study to report poor fracture healing results from NSAIDs when they're used as the primary form of pain relief and in fact, studies on this subject date back to the early 1990s. So how does this equate to LBP? Most directly, fractures are one of the many causes of LBP, so for that population, the answer is clear. However, LBP is much more commonly caused by sprains (ligament injuries) and strains (muscle/tendon injuries), as well as cartilage injury. Here too, studies show that the healing rate of sprains, strains, and cartilage is also delayed when NSAIDs are used as the primary pain relief approach. This healing delay is reportedly due to NSAIDs' inhibition of "proteoglycan synthesis," a component of ligament and cartilage tissue regeneration and repair. NSAIDs also inhibit release of prostaglandins (especially prostaglandin E2), which is needed for tissue repair. These effects are ESPECIALLY observed with long-term use, but recent studies show injured athletes are best off NOT taking NSAIDs AT ALL as these drugs delay the healing process and thus the athlete's ability to return to their sport.

In a January 2015 study, researchers criticized the common use of NSAIDs in elderly patients for the treatment of non-cancerous pain. They found 75% of the elderly population studied was prescribed NSAIDs which, in retrospect, the researchers determined to be inappropriate! Because NSAIDs interfere with healing, the net effect is an ACCELERATION of osteoarthritis and joint deterioration! In 1995, a North Carolina School of Medicine study compared four groups of patients with soft tissue injuries (tendon strains): Group 1 received NO treatment (control group); Group 2 received exercise only; Group 3 received exercise AND Indomethacin; and Group 4 received Indomethacin only. At 72 hours post-injury, ONLY the exercise group had an INCREASE in prostaglandins (E2 particularly – necessary for healing). This effect was even more profound at 108 hours after injury. The research team also found DNA synthesis in the fibroblasts (an important part of the repair mechanism) was greatest in the exercise group and was completely lacking in the NSAID-only group.

Spinal Manipulation for Lumbar Intervertebral Disc Syndrome with Radiculopathy

For thirty years (since 1985), it has been acknowledged that spinal manipulation is successful in the treatment of the majority of patients with low back pain, and that "there is a scientific basis for the treatment of back pain by manipulation." (1) However, the consensus pertaining to the use of spinal manipulation for the treatment of intervertebral disc syndrome with radiculopathy is less investigated. Consequently, there is the potential for an opinion that spinal manipulation may be inappropriate for patients with low back intervertebral disc syndrome and symptoms/signs of radiculopathy. This publication will review a number of articles on this topic, spanning six decades (1954-2015). In 1954, RH Ramsey, MD, published a study titled (2):Conservative Treatment of Intervertebral Disk Lesions. Dr. Ramsey's study appeared in the Instructional Course Lectures of the American Academy of Orthopedic Surgeons . Dr. Ramsey states: "The conservative management of lumbar disk lesions should be given careful consideration because no patient should be considered for surgical treatment without first having failed to respond to an adequate program of conservative treatment." "If after a fair trial of conservative treatment, the pain and disability continue and the symptoms are of sufficient gravity to warrant surgery, the patient is advised that he should be operated upon and the offending disk lesion should be removed."

Dr. Ramsey advocated a number of conservative treatments for this syndrome, including spinal manipulation. Pertaining to manipulation, Dr. Ramsey makes the following comments: "From what is known about the pathology of lumbar disk lesions, it would seem that the ideal form of conservative treatment would theoretically be a manipulative closed reduction of the displaced disk material." "Many forms of manipulation are carried out by orthopedic surgeons and by cultists and this form of treatment will probably always be a controversial one." "We limit the use of manipulation almost entirely to those patients who do not seem to be responding well to non-manipulative conservative treatment and who are anxious to have something else done short of operative intervention." "The patient lies on his side on the edge of the table facing the surgeon and the leg that is up is allowed to drop over the side of the table, tending to swing the up-side of the pelvis forward. The arm that is up is allowed to drop back behind the patient, tending to pull the shoulder back. The surgeon then places one hand on the patient's shoulder and his opposite forearm on the patient's iliac crest. Simultaneously, the shoulder is thrust suddenly back, rotating the torso in one direction while the iliac crest is thrust down and forward, rotating the pelvis in the opposite direction. This gives the lumbar spine a twist that frequently causes an audible and palpable crunch. This procedure is then repeated with the patient on his other side. The patient is then turned on his back and his hips and knees are hyper flexed sufficiently to forcibly flex the lumbar spine which tends to open up the disk spaces posteriorly." "The patient should be cautioned beforehand that forceful manipulation may possibly make his symptoms worse although many patients will get marked relief." Dr. Ramsey notes that the manipulation is "forceful" and associated with an "audible and palpable crunch." Although he cautions that the manipulation may make the patient worse, "many patients will get marked relief."

Fifteen years later (in 1969), physicians JA Mathews and DAH Yates from the Department of Physical Medicine, St. Thomas' Hospital, London, published a study titled (3): Reduction of Lumbar Disc Prolapse by Manipulation This study appeared in the September 20, 1969 issue of the British Medical Journal . These authors evaluated a number of patients that presented with an acute onset of low back and buttock pain that did not respond to rest. Diagnostic epidurography showed a clinically relevant small disc protrusion, along with antalgia and positive lumbar spine nerve stretch tests. These patients were then treated with long-lever rotation manipulations of the lumbar spine, using the shoulder and iliac crest as levers. These lumbar spine manipulations were clearly accompanied with a thrust maneuver. The manipulations were repeated until abnormal symptoms and signs had disappeared. Following the manipulations there was resolution of signs, symptoms, antalgia, and reduction in the size of the protrusions. Drs. Mathews and Yates state: "The frequent accompaniment of acute onset low back pain by spinal deformity suggests a mechanical factor, and the accompanying abnormality of straight-leg raise or femoral stretch test suggests that the lesion impinges on the spinal dura matter of the dural nerve sheaths." "The lumbar spine was rotated away from the painful side to the limit of its range, the buttock or thigh of the painful side being used as a lever; a firm additional thrust was made in the same direction. This manoeuver was repeated until abnormal symptoms and signs had disappeared, progress being assessed by repeated examination." "Rotation manipulations apply torsion stress throughout the lumbar spine. If the posterior longitudinal ligament and the annulus fibrosis are intact, some of this torsion force would tend to exert a centripetal force, reducing prolapsed or bulging disc material."

"The results of this study suggest that small disc protrusions were present in patients presenting with lumbago and that the protrusions were diminished in size when their symptoms had been relieved by manipulations." These authors conclude: "it seems likely that the reduction effect [of the disc protrusion] is due to the manipulating thrust used."

In another study published in 1969, BC Edwards compared the effectiveness of heat/massage/exercise to spinal manipulation in the treatment of 184 patients that were grouped according to the presentation of back and leg pain, as follows (4): Group, Treatment, Acceptable, Outcome Central Low Back Pain Only heat/massage/exercise 83%/spinal manipulation 83%/Pain Radiation to Buttock heat/massage/exercise 70% spinal manipulation 78% Pain Radiation Down Thigh to Knee heat/massage/exercise 65% spinal manipulation 96% Pain Radiation down Leg to Foot heat/massage/exercise 52% spinal manipulation 79%. This study by Edwards was published in the Australian Journal of Physiotherapy . This study by Edwards was reviewed by Augustus A. White, MD, and Manohar M. Panjabi, PhD, in their 1990 book, Clinical Biomechanics of the Spine (5). Drs. White and Panjabi make the following points pertaining to the Edwards article:

"A well-designed, well executed, and well-analyzed study.

"In the group with central low back pain only, "the results were acceptable in 83% for both treatments. However, they were achieved with spinal manipulation using about one-half the number of treatments that were needed for heat, massage, and exercise."

In the group with pain radiating into the buttock, "the results were slightly better with manipulation, and again they were achieved with about half as many treatments."

In the groups with pain radiation to the knee and/or to the foot, "the manipulation therapy was statistically significantly better," and in the group with pain radiating to the foot, "the manipulative therapy is significantly better."

"This study certainly supports the efficacy of spinal manipulative therapy in comparison with heat, massage, and exercise. The results (80 – 95% satisfactory) are impressive in comparison with any form of therapy."

In 1977, the third edition of Orthopedics, Principles and Their Applications was published. The author, Samuel Turek, MD (d. 1986), was a Clinical Professor, Department of Orthopedics and Rehabilitation at the University of Miami School of Medicine. In the section pertaining to the protruded disc, Dr. Turek makes the following observations (6): Treatment of Intervertebral Disc Herniation With Manipulation

"Manipulation. Some orthopedic surgeons practice manipulation in an effort at repositioning the disc. This treatment is regarded as controversial and a form of quackery by many men. However, the author has attempted the maneuver in patients who did not respond to bed rest and were regarded as candidates for surgery. Occasionally, the results were dramatic.

Technique. The patient lies on his side on the edge of the table facing the surgeon, and the uppermost leg is allowed to drop forward over the edge of the table, carrying forward that side of the pelvis. The uppermost arm is placed backward behind the patient, pulling the shoulder back. The surgeon places one hand on the shoulder and the other on the iliac crest and twists the torso by pushing the shoulder backward and the iliac crest forward. The maneuver is sudden and forceful and frequently is associated with an audible and palpable crunching sound in the lower back. When this is felt, the relief of pain is usually immediate. The maneuver is repeated with the patient on the opposite side."

"The patient should be cautioned beforehand that the manipulation may make his symptoms worse and that this is an attempt to avoid surgery."

In February 1987, physicians Paul Pang-Fu Kuo and Zhen-Chao Loh published an important study pertaining to lumbar disc protrusions and rotary spinal manipulation, titled (7):

Treatment of Lumbar Intervertebral Disc Protrusions by Manipulation

Their article appeared in the journal Clinical Orthopedics and Related Research . Drs. Paul Pang-Fu Kuo and Zhen-Chao Loh are from the Department of Orthopedic Surgery, Shanghai Second Medical College, and Chief Surgeon, Department of Orthopaedic Surgery,

Rui Jin Hospital, Shanghai, China. They note that manipulation has been used in Chinese healthcare for thousands of years, and by the Tang Dynasty (618-907 AD), who noted "manipulation was fully established and became a routine for the treatment of low back pain."

In their study, they performed a series of eight manipulations on 517 patients with protruded lumbar discs and clinically relevant signs and symptoms. Their outcomes were quite good, with 84% achieving a successful outcome and only 9% not responding. Only 14 % suffered a reoccurrence of symptoms at intervals ranging from two months to twelve years. These authors state:

"The patient is placed on the sound side first with the hip and knee of the painful side flexed and the sound side straight. The operator rests one hand in front of the shoulder and the other hand on the buttock. By simultaneously pulling the shoulder backwards and pushing the buttock forwards, a snap or click can usually be heard or felt. This manipulation may then be repeated on the other side as required."

"Manipulation of the spine can be effective treatment for lumbar disc protrusions."

"Most protruded discs may be manipulated. When the diagnosis is in doubt, gentle force should be used at first as a trial in order to gain the confidence of the patient."

"During manipulation a snap may accompany rotation. Subjectively it has dramatic influence on both patient and operator and is thought to be a sign of relief."

"If derangement of the facets or subluxation of the posterior elements near the protruded disc occurs, the rotation may have caused reduction, giving remarkable relief."

"Gapping of the disc on bending and rotation may create a condition favorable for the possible reentry of the protruded disc into the intervertebral cavity, or the rotary manipulation may cause the protruded disc to shift away from pressing on the nerve root."

In terms of applying manipulation, Drs. Kuo and Loh indicate "practice is necessary to become proficient in spinal manipulation techniques," and "expertise plays an important role in the success of manipulation." The manipulation of disc protrusions should be performed only by trained experts. Additionally, manipulation is contraindicated if the patient is suffering from incontinence or paraplegia.

In 1989, the Journal of Manipulative and Physiological Therapeutics published a case study of a patient with an "enormous central herniation lumbar disc" who underwent a course of side posture manipulation (8). The patient improved considerably with only 2 weeks of treatment. The authors state:

"It is emphasized that manipulation has been shown to be an effective treatment for some patients with lumbar disc herniation.

While complications of this form of treatment have been reported in the literature, such incidents are rare."

In 1993, chiropractor J. David Cassidy, chiropractor Haymo Thiel, and physician (orthopedic surgeon) William Kirkaldy-Willis published a "Review Of The Literature" article titled (9):

Side posture manipulation for lumbar intervertebral disk herniation

These authors are from the Department of Orthopedics, Royal University Hospital, Saskatoon, Saskatchewan, Canada, and their article appeared in the Journal of Manipulative and Physiological Therapeutics .

In their article, these authors cite studies on human cadavers that show the annulus of the disc is quite resistant to rotational stresses. Specifically, a normal disc did not show failure until 22.6° of rotational stress, and a degenerated disc could withstand an average of 14.3° of rotational stress. They therefore conclude "torsional failure of the lumbar disk first requires fracture of the posterior joints" before there is any annular tearing.

When performing rotational manipulation in the management of lumbar disc herniation, these authors suggest that it is wise to begin with mobilization prior to performing manipulation to assess the patient's responses. Additionally, they state that if positioning increases leg pain, "one should not proceed to manipulation at that particular session."

Based upon their review of the literature and their own experiences, these authors state:

"The treatment of lumbar disk herniation by side posture manipulation is not new and has been advocated by both chiropractors and medical manipulators."

"The treatment of lumbar intervertebral disk herniation by side posture manipulation is both safe and effective."

In 1995, chiropractors PJ Stern, Peter Côté P, and David Cassidy published a study titled (10):

A series of consecutive cases of low back pain with radiating leg pain treated by chiropractors

Their article appeared in the Journal of Manipulative and Physiological Therapeutics . The authors retrospectively reviewed the outcomes of 59 consecutive patients complaining of low back and radiating leg pain, and were clinically diagnosed as having a lumbar spine disk herniation. Ninety percent of these patients reported improvement of their complaint after chiropractic manipulation. The maximum complication rate associated with this treatment approach was estimated to be 5% or less. A previous history of low back surgery was a statistically significant predictor of poor outcome. They concluded:

"Based on our results, we postulate that a course of non-operative treatment including manipulation may be effective   and safe for the treatment of back and radiating leg pain."

In 2006, physicians Valter Santilli, MD, Ettore Beghi, MD, Stefano Finucci, MD, published an article in The Spine Journal titled (11):

Chiropractic manipulation in the treatment of acute back pain and sciatica with disc protrusion:
A randomized double-blind clinical trial of active and simulated spinal manipulations

The purpose of this study was to assess the short- and long-term effects of spinal manipulations on acute back pain and sciatica with disc protrusion. It is a randomized double-blind trial comparing active and simulated manipulations for these patients. The study used 102 patients. The manipulations or simulated manipulations were done 5 days per week by experienced chiropractors for up to a maximum of 20 patient visits, "using a rapid thrust technique." Re-evaluations were done at 15, 30, 45, 90, and 180 days.

The authors list rationales for using manipulation in the treatment of low back pain and sciatica to include:

- Reduction of a bulging disc
- Correction of disc displacement
- Release of adhesive fibrosis surrounding prolapsed discs or facet joints
- Release of entrapped synovial folds
- Inhibition of nociceptive impulses
- Relaxation of hypertonic muscles
- Unbuckling displaced motion segments

The authors noted the following observations:

"Active manipulations have more effect than simulated manipulations on pain relief for acute back pain and sciatica with disc protrusion."

"At the end of follow-up a significant difference was present between active and simulated manipulations in the percentage of cases becoming pain-free (local pain 28% vs. 6%; radiating pain 55% vs. 20%)."

"Patients receiving active manipulations enjoyed significantly greater relief of local and radiating acute LBP, spent fewer days with moderate-to-severe pain, and consumed fewer drugs for the control of pain."

"No adverse events were reported."

The authors concluded that chiropractic spinal "manipulations may relieve acute back pain and sciatica with disc protrusion."

Real Manipulations

Simulated Manipulations

# of Subjects 53 49% of Local Pain Free Subjects 28% 6% % of Radiation Pain Free Subjects 55% 20%

In 2014, an interdisciplinary group of physicians, chiropractors, and researchers published a study in the Annals of Internal Medicine, titled (12):

Spinal Manipulation and Home Exercise With Advice for Subacute and Chronic Back-Related Leg Pain

This study was funded by the United States Department of Health and Human Services. It included 192 patients who were suffering from back-related leg pain for least 4 weeks. The number of subjects in the study gave it good statistical power. The subjects were randomized into either:

- Chiropractic spinal manipulation + home exercise and advice, or
- Home exercise and advice alone

The treatment lasted 12 weeks. The authors concluded:

"For leg pain, spinal manipulative therapy plus home exercise and advice had a clinically important advantage over home exercise and advice (difference, 10 percentage points) at 12 weeks."

"Spinal manipulative therapy with home exercise and advice improved self-reported pain and function outcomes more than exercise and advice alone at 12 weeks."

"Spinal manipulative therapy combined with home exercise and advice can improve short-term outcomes in patients with back-related leg pain."

"For patients with subacute and chronic back-related leg pain, spinal manipulative therapy in addition to home exercise and advice is a safe and effective conservative treatment approach,   resulting in better short-term outcomes than home exercise and   advice alone."

"No serious treatment-related adverse events or deaths occurred."

In another 2014 study, a group of multidisciplinary researchers and chiropractic clinicians from Switzerland presented a prospective study involving 148 patients with low back and leg pain. The study was published in the Journal of Manipulative and Physiological Therapeutics and titled (13):

Outcomes of Acute and Chronic Patients with Magnetic Resonance Imaging–Confirmed Symptomatic Lumbar Disc Herniations Receiving High-Velocity, Low-Amplitude, Spinal Manipulative Therapy:

A Prospective Observational Cohort Study With One-Year Follow-Up

The purpose of this study was to document outcomes of patients with confirmed, symptomatic lumbar disc herniations and sciatica that were treated with chiropractic side posture high-velocity, low-amplitude, spinal manipulation to the level of the disc herniation. It is important to emphasize that all patients in this study had clear abnormal physical examination findings of radiculopathy, including positive MRI abnormalities that corresponded with their symptoms and physical findings. Their pain was rated using the numerical rating scale and their disability was measured with the Oswestry questionnaire. Evaluations were performed at 2 weeks, 1 month, 3 months, 6 months, and 12 months.

The outcomes from this study are summarized in the following table:

Substantial Improvement (rounded)

2 weeks

1 month

3 months

6 months

12 months

Entire group

70% 80% 91% 89% 88%

Acute group

81% 85% 95% 91% 86%

Chronic group

47% 71% 82% 89% 89%

The authors make the following statements:

"The proportion of patients reporting clinically relevant improvement in this current study is surprisingly good, with nearly 70% of patients improved as early as 2 weeks after the start of treatment. By 3 months, this figure was up to 90.5% and then stabilized at 6 months and 1 year."

"A large percentage of acute and importantly chronic lumbar disc herniation patients treated with chiropractic spinal manipulation reported clinically relevant improvement."

"Even the chronic patients in this study, with the mean duration of their symptoms being over 450 days, reported significant improvement, although this takes slightly longer."

"A large percentage of acute and importantly chronic lumbar disc herniation patients treated with high-velocity, low- amplitude side posture spinal manipulative therapy reported clinically relevant 'improvement' with no serious adverse events."

"Spinal Manipulative therapy is a very safe and cost-effective option for treating symptomatic lumbar disc herniation."

This study shows that patients with proven lumbar intervertebral disc herniation and compressive neuropathology that receive traditional chiropractic side-posture manipulation is both safe and effective. The ultimate clinical effectiveness of about 90% is impressive when compared to any form of therapy, and with no reported serious side effects.

This study would suggest that all patients suffering from lumbar intervertebral disc herniation with compressive neuropathology should be treated with chiropractic spinal adjusting.

Who Gets Low Back Pain?

Low back pain (LBP) occurs all over the world. Between 2004 and 2008, an estimated 2.06 million EPISODES of LBP occurred in the United States (US) alone! Each year, LBP accounts for 3.15% of all emergency visits with 65% of LB injuries occurring at home. According to estimates, two-thirds of all Americans will experience at least one episode of back pain during their lifetime. Interestingly, according to one study, LBP peaks two times during life: between 25-29 years of age and 95-99 years of age, regardless of cause. Looking at gender differences, when analyzed by five year age groups, males aged 10-49 and females aged 65-94 had a greater risk for LBP when compared with the opposite gender. Those with European or African ancestry have significantly higher rates of LBP when compared with those of Asian ancestry. Also, older patients have the greatest risk of hospital admission for LBP.

In order to study the incidence of LBP among active duty US military service members, a 2012 study investigated the US Defense Medical Epidemiology Database and looked at 13,754,261 person-years of data (100 25-year-olds would equal 2,500 person-years, for example). The authors of the study report that women have a 45% higher incidence rate than men, and personnel over age 40 are 1.28 times more likely to experience back pain than those who are 25-29 years old. Looking at single vs. married service members, married personnel have a higher incidence rate (1.21) than non-married personnel, though there is no consensus as to why this is the case. In conclusion, the female gender, age >40 years, and those who are married have the greater risk for LBP in the military.

One study looked at alcohol consumption and the incidence of LBP to see if there was a causal relationship between the two. After searching the literature, no positive link between alcohol consumption and LBP was found. On the other hand, smoking clearly contributes to the incidence of LBP (yet another reason to quit smoking!). One study looked at daily use, number of years smoked, and total cigarette use during the years of smoking in relation to LBP in 29,424 monozygotic (identical) twin pairs where only one of the two twins smoked. Researchers determined how many days in the past year LBP was present (1-7 days, 8-30 days, and >30 days) and age, gender, and size/body mass index for each participant. The results revealed a positive association with smoking and the duration of LBP at 1-7 days (1.4 odds ratio), 8-30 days (2.1), and >30 days (3.0) during the past year.

Back Pain Relief in Just One Visit?

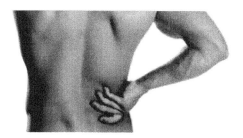

Lacey / Olympia WA – If you suffer with back pain and would like to find relief as quickly as possible…this might be the most important thing you ever read.

In just a moment, I'm going to tell you about a back pain treatment that has gained recent popularity for some very good reasons.

But first – let me ask you this…

What would it be worth to you if you could ends your back pain with just one 20 minute visit to a local doctor right here in Lacey / Olympia?

How would it make you feel if you could do all the things you want and love to do – without back pain?

Sadly, there is no back pain treatment that can guarantee results like that. In fact, there is no back pain treatment that can guarantee any results what-so-ever.

That's not how it works in the real world. SO, if you are looking for an "instant miracle cure," this is not for you.

But, if you are looking for a great back pain treatment that has already helped countless others possibly just like you – with the quality scientific research to back it up – this is perfect for you.

Here is why: Dr. David Warwick is a Chiropractor right here in Lacey. You probably know about Chiropractors – but here is something you probably do not know.
Dr. Warwick has a very busy practice for two reasons…

First are results. Dr. Warwick uses only mainstream, scientifically researched techniques that give patients the best chance to get out of pain as fast as possible.

What results can be expected?
Here is what a 2014 study published in Journal of Manipulative and Physiological Therapeutics said about one of the treatments Dr. Warwick uses:
"The proportion of patients reporting clinically relevant improvement in this current study is surprisingly good, with nearly 70% of patients improved as early as 2 weeks after the start of treatment. By 3 months, this figure was up to 90.5% and then stabilized at 6 months and 1 year."

Those are some great results, but you must understand this: Because every case is individual, it is impossible to predict results.
And here is something Dr. Warwick does his patients absolutely love.

Dr. Warwick does not make his patients commit to any long term, expensive treatment programs. Instead, he offers, treatment one visit at a time – without any obligation or commitment.

That is why Dr. Warwick offers a **free consultation** where you get all your questions answered and you find out if you qualify for his treatments. Of course, there is never any obligation of commitment. If you would like a free consultation to see if Dr. Warwick can help you – or if you have any questions, just call **360-951-4504** or schedule an appointment with Dr. David Warwick

What's Causing My Back Pain?

Low back pain (LBP) is one of the most common reasons patients seek out Chiropractic care, and they appreciate being told what is causing their back pain. This is why doctors gather a careful and complete history from new patients and perform a physical examination. Once the "pain generator" is determined, a doctor can discuss various treatment options and develop a plan for managing the patient. Let's review some causes of LBP!

If we divide the various conditions into three categories, it significantly improves diagnostic accuracy. These include: 1) Mechanical LBP; 2) Nerve root pain; and 3) "Red Flags" (serious conditions). The most common conditions are those belonging to the first group. The following is a partial list of conditions that belong to each category:

1. Mechanical LBP: Causes of mechanical LBP include Lumbar and sacroiliac (SI) sprains, lumbar muscle strains, facet syndrome, degenerative disk disease (DDD) and/or injury to the disk without nerve pinch, osteoarthritis (this can affect different parts of the spine), spinal instability, spondylolysis and/or spondylolisthesis, and more. The pain pattern is usually localized to the low back and may spread into the buttocks, hips, thighs, but rarely extends past the knee. Usually, there is NO numbness or weakness in the leg or foot because that symptom suggests a spinal nerve pinch.
2. Nerve root pain can result from herniated disk (from either direct nerve pinching and/or chemical irritation inflaming the nerve), central or lateral spinal stenosis (usually caused by a combination of things including DDD), arthritis, and/or calcification of ligaments near the nerve. These can be managed very successfully without surgery but the careful monitoring of numbness, muscle weakness, and treatment satisfaction is important!
3. Red Flags: These are the potentially dangerous conditions such as cancer, fracture, infections, cauda equina syndrome (spinal cord pinch creating bowel and/or bladder weakness). Referred pain from organs may be included here as well. As you

can see, these carry potentially lethal consequences and require immediate referral and specialty management.

The majority of patients suffering from LBP fall into the first two categories, and the HISTORY can tell us a lot! If the patient complains of pain that stays mostly in the low back but may spread into the buttocks or thigh without numbness/weakness in the leg and feels better with leaning forwards or curling up in a ball, it probably is a Group 1 (mechanical) diagnosis. If there is numbness, tingling, and/or weakness in the leg to the foot and bending over hurts, it's most likely disk derangement (bulge, herniated, etc.) with a nerve pinch. If there is unexplained weight loss, a past history of cancer, non-responding LBP to treatment, sleep interruptions, and age >50 years old, we may now be in category three and further tests are needed!

The IMPORTANT point is that spinal manipulation (chiropractic) can manage the most common causes of LBP as a non-surgical, low-risk form of care.

Low Back Pain – What To Do & NOT Do!

Low back pain (LBP) can strike at any time or place, often when we least expect it. There are "self-help" approaches that can be of great benefit, but many of these approaches can fail, or worse, irritate the condition. Here are some "do's and don'ts" when self-managing low back pain!

Ice vs. Heat? Typically, people are almost always confused about which is better, ice or heat? This decision can be significantly helpful or hurtful, depending on the case. Generally, "ice is nice," as it vasoconstricts and pushes out inflammation or swelling, which usually feels relieving and helpful even though the initial "shock" of ice may not be too appealing to most of us! This is probably why MOST people will wrongly choose heat as their initial course of self-care.

This is usually wrong because heat vasodilates, which draws blood into the injured area that is already inflamed and swollen, thus adding more fluid to the injured area — sort of like throwing gas on a fire! Heat may feel good initially, but often soon after, increased pain intensity and frequency may occur. When LBP is chronic or NOT new / acute, heat can be very helpful, as it relaxes muscles and improves movement by reducing stiffness (but never use heat more than 20 minutes per hour).

The biggest mistake about the use of heat is leaving it on too long – some people even burn themselves with a heating pad they've left on for hours of continuous use – sometimes overnight (PLEASE DON'T DO THAT!). When using ice, there are MANY ways one can apply it. If you only have 5-10 minutes, that is better than nothing! However, an ideal approach is to apply the ice pack or bag as follows: On 15 min. / off 15 min. / on 15 min. / off 15 min. / on 15 minutes (total time: 1:15 hr.). The "off 15 minutes" helps the area to warm up by allowing the blood to come back into the low back area, which avoids frost bite and sets up a pump-like action.

Even better is an approach called "CONTRAST THERAPY" where we start and end with ice and use heat in between as follows: ICE 10 minutes / HEAT 5 min. / ICE 10 min. / HEAT 5 min. / ICE 10 min. (total time: 40 minutes). This approach creates a stronger pump-like or "push-pull" action that pushes out fluids/inflammation (with ice) followed by pulling in fluids (with heat). Both approaches are effective! If you ever feel worse after icing, PLEASE STOP AND CONTACT US, as you may have a unique case or situation.

How active should I be? Here too, most people usually try to do too much even after they feel "warning signs". It's human nature to want to "…get things done," so sometimes we push ourselves beyond the limits of our tissue's capacity, resulting in an injury. Once we've hurt our back, we STILL try to stay with our daily routine, ignoring our LBP the best we can. Generally, it's BETTER to be a little active than it is to be too sedentary, but there is also a limit, as too much activity is like "…picking at a cut," only prolonging healing and recovery.

If every time you bend over results in a sharp, dagger-like pain in your low back, PLEASE STOP and assess the situation! Position preference is the KEY to determining what type of stretches or other exercises may be best for you. So, if bending over REDUCES LBP, pull your knees to your chest (we'll show you how)! If bending backwards feels better, we'll show you several extension exercises that can be done multiple times a day. Remember, too much sitting or lying down will weaken your low back muscles. Emphasize positions that feel good and avoid sharp, lancinating pain!

Chiropractic Care and X-Rays for Low Back Pain

Low back pain (LBP) is the most common complaint for which patients seek chiropractic care. X-rays are a common diagnostic tool utilized by most health care providers. Let's take a look at the role of x-rays and how they are used by both medical practitioners and chiropractors.

X-rays are a form of radiation (similar to light or radio waves) that focuses a beam on a subject such as a person or specific body part. The x-rays mostly pass through softer tissues while hard tissues like teeth and bones do not allow the beam to pass through, which leaves a "white" image on the film. More dense soft tissues, like muscles and organs, will appear as various shades of gray while less dense areas, like the lungs or bowel, will appear black on an x-ray.

Spinal x-rays are basically pictures of the spine that are taken to help the doctor determine a diagnosis as to the cause of the patient's particular problem. Typically, a patient provides a medical history and the doctor performs a clinical examination to establish a primary diagnosis. When necessary, the doctor may order diagnostic tests like x-ray (or a CT, MRI, bone scan, PET scan, ultrasound, blood tests, tissue biopsy, and so on) in attempt to verify or validate the diagnosis. Spinal x-rays include the bony spine, the disk spaces (between each vertebra – but not the actual disk), and often the pelvis (with or without the hip joints), and extend up to the lower thoracic spine where the lower few ribs are located, depending on the patient's height. Usually, frontal and side views are taken. Other views may include a "spot" (close up), obliques, or flexion/extension stress views. So, what are we looking for?

The FIRST order of business is to make sure we're not dealing with something potentially dangerous like fractures, infections, dislocations, tumors/cancer, and so forth. We look for other things like bone spurs ("osteoarthritis"), the disk heights (disks narrow as they degenerate, usually accompanied with bone spurs), joint spaces, bone density, and alignment – like scoliosis. Chiropractors typically take spinal x-rays in a weight-bearing position (standing) while most medical facilities take their x-rays with the patient lying down. The "pro" of a weight bearing x-ray is the ability to measure for things like scoliosis, leg length deficiency (a short leg), and joint space narrowing favoring the standing approach. The "con" of weight-bearing x-ray is something called "movement artifact" or, a blurred image. Recumbent films tend to be clearer and more detailed but with less of an ability to accurately take measurements to evaluate things like leg length or the extent of spinal misalignment. Both MD's and DC's take scoliosis films standing, but otherwise, MD's favor laying down x-rays while DC's favor standing. Regarding the "safety vs. harm" factor of taking an x-ray or not, most guidelines favor waiting if there is no suspicion of pathology (cancer, fracture, infection, etc.) for both professions. However, when a significant biomechanical problem is suspected, especially if a treatment decision is driven by the test's outcome, it may be appropriate to take x-rays. For example, the use of heel lifts to correct a short leg is also measured on the x-ray. There are also some chiropractic techniques that rely on assessing the bony alignment, which include taking measurements from an x-ray as well. Patient safety is first and each case must be individually assessed. If you think you may be pregnant, DO NOT LET ANYONE X-RAY YOU!

Low Back Pain in the Older Adult

Last month, we addressed low back pain (LBP) in the younger patient (age 30-60), so it only seems appropriate to continue the discussion for those over the age of 60. As previously mentioned, back pain does NOT discriminate when it comes to age. In fact, chiropractors see many children and teenagers with LBP as well as 90+ year-olds! Let's take a look at the "usual" differences...

In the younger adult, facet syndrome and disk derangement are common conditions, and though this can still occur in the older adult, it becomes less common after age 60. The primary reason is because our disks become dehydrated or "dry up" as we age, making them less likely to herniate compared to a young, well-hydrated disk. During this "dehydration" process, the disks gradually narrow and bulge outwards. Therefore, in the 60+ year-old adult, disk-related pain is typically NOT from the soft liquid center herniating through the tough outer "annular" layer as it does in the younger patient. Rather, it's from a combination of conditions. These conditions combine together and result in narrowing of the openings through which the nerve root exits the spine (called the neuroforamen).

The multiple conditions that contribute to this process include (but are not limited to): narrowing and bulging of the disk, osteoarthritis, or spurring extending off the vertebral endplates where the disk attaches, facet joint arthritis resulting in "hypertrophy" or enlargement, calcification of ligaments, and more. WHEN the neuroforamen narrows to the point of pinching the nerve root, symptoms occur. This condition is called "spinal stenosis" (SS), which literally means, "narrowed spinal canals" with entrapment of the spinal cord and/or nerves. Classic symptoms associated with SS include low back pain and stiffness. Most importantly, SS causes a gradual reduction in the amount of time that people with this condition can tolerate walking. Restricted mobility is initially subtle, but after months and years, walking may become more and more limited. That is, every time a certain time frame is reached (like 5 or 10 minutes of walking), the symptoms become significant to the point they force the SS patient to stop and sit or bend over often for one to two minutes, after which time they are able to resume walking for a similar amount of time.

Another common feature is that bending forwards HELPS (because it opens up the neuroforamen), and many SS patients walk bent over as their "norm." When walking in a grocery store, they may lean forwards on the grocery cart because it allows for a longer, less painful walk. Other symptoms common with osteoarthritis (which always precedes SS), include morning stiffness, stiffness and pain when rising from sitting, decreased range of spinal motion or flexibility, localized painful joints, and others. As mentioned previously, degenerative joint disease or osteoarthritis is a slow, smoldering process that can often be traced back over the past 5, 10, and even 20 years.

As chiropractors, we can improve spinal joint flexibility and slow this process down. Give chiropractic a try as back pain in our elderly years DOES NOT have to be disabling!

Low Back Pain and Younger Adults

Low back pain (LBP) is so common that if you haven't had it by now, you will! Let's take a look at some the possible causes of LBP and what we might be able to do when LBP strikes.

Typically, younger individuals are NOT immune to LBP. In fact, those between 30-60 years of age are MORE likely to experience LBP caused from a muscle strain, ligament sprain, or disk "derangement" such as a herniated disk. Here are some specific causes:

LBP from a sudden movement or lifting a heavy object – Typical symptoms include: a) Difficulty moving that can be so severe it can prevent walking or standing. b) Pain that does NOT radiate down the leg past the knee but may refer pain into the groin, buttock, or upper thigh. c) Pain that tends to be achy and dull. d) Muscle spasms (that can be severe). e) Local soreness noted upon touch. DIAGNOSIS: The most likely injuries described by the scenario above include a muscle strain or ligament sprain (or, a muscle or ligament pull/stretch/tear that can break down into mild vs. moderate vs. severe, or, microscopic tears vs. up to 75% tearing vs. >75% tearing may occur, respectively). The severity of the injury and how well you take care of yourself will determine healing time. TREATMENT can include Chiropractic care, ice (15 min. rotations on/off/on/off/on), activity modifications (usually, a combination of walking and resting for the first day or two will help but after that, we will guide you in the proper exercises for stretching and eventually strengthening), and anti-inflammatory care. We prefer herbs such as ginger, turmeric, boswellia, and other nutrients over NSAIDs — like Advil, Aleve, and aspirin — as these irritate the stomach and can damage the liver and kidney. Recent studies show that NSAIDs can also inhibit important chemical activities in the body that may actually slow the healing process. For this reason, studies have concluded that athletes who are trying to get back into their sport should be advised NOT to take NSAIDs! The same should apply to everyone, don't you think?

LBP that travels past the knee down the back of the leg often to the ankle or foot is frequently referred to as sciatica. This may include: a) Pain that is longer lasting rather than flaring up for a few days or one to two weeks. b) Pain may be greater in the leg than the low back. c) Pain is commonly on one side. d) Pain is worsened by sitting and or bending forwards, and improved by standing and or bending backwards. e) Symptoms often includes pain, in addition to numbness/tingling, and/or burning. f) Muscle shrinkage and weakness on the involved side may occur as well. DIAGNOSIS: In this age group, lumbar herniated disk (LDH) is the most likely cause. The lower two disks – L4/5 and L5/S1 — are the two most common locations for herniated disks. The odd thing about LDH's is that about 50% of us have bulging disks and 20% of us have herniated disks but have NO pain! TREATMENT: Try chiropractic first. It works and you can always have surgery later, but you can't go back after it's done! We will refer you if our approaches are not satisfying!

Back Pain Relief – The Most Important Factor?

What every back pain sufferer should know before choosing a doctor or starting *any* back pain treatment.

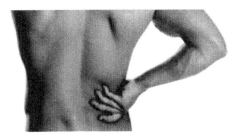

Lacey / Olympia – There is no doubt. Back pain is life changing. Nothing is worse than being in constant pain – and not being able to do all the things you once could. And just as bad as the pain is the frustration of not being able to find a solution.

How would you like to finally find a solution for your back pain? A solution that is 100% guaranteed to work and cure your back pain...instantly?

The bad news is – there is no "100% guaranteed cure" for back pain. And no ethical doctor would make such a claim. Real, ethical doctors use a scientific research and do not make ridiculous claims. In other words, they are honest and up front with patients and give them the best options possible and are honest about the possible outcomes.

The good news – there are some wonderful treatments for back pain that often get great results. And because no one treatment works for everyone – the key is to find what treatment is right for your individual case.

That can be the difference between finally relieving your pain and continuing to suffer.

That's why the most important factor in finding relief for your back pain is choosing the right doctor. That may seem obvious – but it is not what you think. Here is why...

It is important to find a doctor that is "mainstream." This means they are knowledgeable about treatments that are scientifically based. It also means that they are well respected by their colleagues and actively refer to other doctors.

The most important thing is the doctor you choose should be "patient centered." This means he or she always finds out what you want – and gives it to you.

Because this is so important a large group of Chiropractic Physicians have taken an amazing pledge in an effort to let patients know what kind of care you can expect.

These doctors are member of ChiroTrust and here is their pledge "To the best of my ability, I agree to provide my patients convenient, affordable, mainstream Chiropractic care. I will not use unnecessary long-term treatment plans and/or therapies."

In other words, if you choose a ChiroTrust doctor you can expect to get the best possible care and the doctor will try to get you better as soon as possible and out of the office.

In fact, ChiroTrust doctors do not offer multiple visit plans and will see you one visit at a time. Patients usually breathe a big sigh of relief because there is no commitment and they get to try out treatments and see if they like them.

And just as important – this makes treatment very affordable for patients without insurance coverage.

Here is something you need to know: ChiroTrust doctors do not just treat you by themselves in isolation. They have great relationships with other doctors in the community and will work with them to get you the best possible care for your individual case.

In other words, you will be going to a trusted advisor who will help you get exactly what you want.

If this sounds great and you would like to see if a ChiroTrust doctor can help your back pain – you are going to love this...

Dr. David Warwick is a ChiroTrust doctor and his practice is off Marvin and Martin right here in Lacey. He offers a limited amount of free consultations every month and if you would like one just call **360-951-4504** or **Walk In**. Consultations are limited due to time constraints because Dr. Warwick always makes sure he has the time necessary for each and every patient. At the consultation you will get all your questions answered and given the best options to help your back pain. Of course there is no obligation and it is completely free. **Contact** Dr. David Warwick today!

Two Important, Yet Simple Tests for Low Back Pain / Leg Pain

The nervous system can be categorized in many different ways. In understanding nervous system physiology, a simple but accurate way of categorization is to view the nervous system as two separate but integrated systems:

- The MOTOR nerve system
- The SENSORY nerve system

The MOTOR nervous system is the nerves that move our muscles (motor), and also control the function of our visceral organs (like heart, lungs, intestines, pancreas, liver, kidneys, etc.). The nerves that send the electrical signal from our brain and spinal cord to our muscles to control their contraction are actually called motor nerves. The nerves that send the electrical signal from our brain and spinal cord to control the function of our visceral organs are called autonomic nerves. This is because they function automatically, without our thinking and even when we are sleeping. Occasionally these autonomic visceral organ nerves are called visceral motor nerves.
The motor nerve systems are output nerves, also called efferent nerves.

The SENSORY nerve system is the nerves that send electrical nerve signals into our spinal cord and brain. Therefore, the sensory nerves travel in the opposite direction of the motor nerves. The sensory nerve systems are input nerves, also called afferent nerves.

The sensory nerves have special endings (receptors) that can take environmental events, convert these events into an electrical signal, and send the electrical signal along sensory nerves to the brain for interpretation. The sensory nerves create our senses. It is our lifelong sensory experiences that "mold" our brain.

There are six primary sensory inputs into our brains:

- Sight (vision). Our eye has specific sensory receptors that have the ability to take specific electromagnetic waves in the environment, convert them into an electrical signal, send the electrical signal along a nerve (the optic nerve) to a specific place in the brain for interpretation (the occipital visual cortex).
- Sound (hearing). Similarly, the ear has specific sensory receptors that have the ability to take specific environmental disturbances, convert them into an electrical signal, send the electrical signal along a nerve (cochlear nerve) to a specific place in the brain for interpretation (the superior gyrus of the temporal lobe).
- Taste. When molecules from food or drink contact our tongue, again an electrical signal is sent via a sensory nerve to the brain for interpretation.
- Smell. When certain molecules in the air travel up our nose, an electrical signal is again sent via a sensory nerve to the brain for interpretation.
- Touch (requires sub categorization). There are special receptors on our skin and in other tissues like muscle, tongue, teeth, and viscera that generate an electrical single when they are mechanically perturbed. This electrical signal is once again sent via sensory nerves to the appropriate place in the brain for interpretation.

- Proprioception. Proprioception is often referred to as our "sixth" sense. There are special receptors in our skin, muscles, joints, fascia, etc., that generate an electrical signal that lets the brain know where we are in space. These receptors and their sensory nerves inform the brain about changes in the position and movements of the various parts of our bodies. Most of us know where our nose is, even when our eyes are closed, and we can easily touch our nose with the tip of our index finger (we also know where the tip of our finger is, even with eyes closed). With our eyes closed, we cannot see, hear, smell, taste, or touch our nose or fingertip, yet we can easily connect the two. This is proprioception.

Touch (#5) requires elaboration. Touch (for our purposes) will also include the sensations of pain and temperature (hot/cold). When there is a perturbation on our skin, we readily can distinguish between touch, pain, hot, and/or cold. All of these sensations are electrical signals that travel to various parts of the brain for interpretation.

The important point is that all perceptions (sight, sound, taste, smell, touch [including pain and temperature] and proprioception) occur in the cortical brain. "All perceptions are cortical." This means that they occur in our brain. Lay people often believe that their eye sees, their ear hears, their tongue tastes, their nose smells, or that something at their toe or back or neck hurts. But actually these various parts of our body only initiate an electrical signal that is then interpreted in our brain.

The cortical perception of pain is a universal human experience. The electrical signal for the perception of pain in the brain is brought to the brain via special sensory nerves called nociceptive afferents or nociceptors .

All sensory inputs into the brain begin with a special receptor, except for pain (nociception). The receptor that initiates the electrical signal for sight is different than the receptor that initiates the electrical signal for sound or taste or smell. Pain (nociception) is the great receptor exception in that, for the most part, there is no receptor on the end of the nociceptive nerves. Consequently, the nociceptive nerve beginnings are referred to as free or naked receptors.

The pain problem in our country (USA) and in the world is astonishingly huge and it is getting worse. In the United States alone, 116 million Americans suffer from chronic daily pain (1). A recent cover article in the newspaper The Wall Street Journal quantifies the anatomical regions for American's chronic pain (2):

Hip Pain	07.1%
Finger Pain	07.6%
Shoulder Pain	09.0%
Neck Pain	15.1%
Severe Headache	16.1%
Knee Pain	19.5%
Lower-Back Pain	28.1%

The total cost attributed to America's pain problem, including treatment, lost productivity, and disability, is approaching $1 trillion per year.

It is useful to discuss pain using the categorizations of C. Chan Gunn, MD (3, 4). Dr. Gunn is a Clinical Professor at the Multidisciplinary Pain Center at the University of Washington Medical School, Seattle, Washington. Dr. Gunn's pain categories are:

1) Nociception Pain

In this category of pain, there is no tissue damage, and therefore no inflammation. This is the type of pain one would experience if someone stepped on your toe; one would have pain but no tissue damage or inflammation. This type of pain does not require a healthcare provider to diagnose the cause of the pain. The cause of the pain is obvious; someone is standing on your toe.

Likewise, this type of pain does not require healthcare provider treatment. The treatment is obvious; get the person's foot off your toe. The patient self-treats.

With this type of pain, once the person's foot is off your toe, you experience immediate and lasting relief. The prognosis is excellent.

This is the type of pain that most patients (and insurance companies) hope they are experiencing, hoping for instant relief. Sadly, this type of pain rarely makes it into a doctor's office because it is self-diagnosed and treated.

2) Algogenic Pain

Suppose that instead of someone stepping on your toe, they smacked your toe with a sledgehammer. Even though the hammer is no longer actually on your toe, your toe still hurts. The hammer added something to the equation, trauma, tissue damage, and inflammation. This disruption of the tissues and blood vessels by the trauma produces and releases inflammatory chemicals that are often collectively called algogenic exudates .

The inflammatory algogenic chemicals alter the thresholds of the nociceptive afferent system , increasing the pain electrical signal to the brain. Instant relief for this type of pain is not possible. The pain subsides as inflammation resolves and the nociceptive afferents system becomes sub-threshold.

Individuals suffering from this type of pain often go to healthcare providers for relief. Treatment often involves anti-inflammatory efforts (controlled motion, drugs, omega-3s, ice, electrical modalities, low–level laser therapy, etc.) and efforts to accelerate healing (low-level laser therapy). Depending upon the degree of tissue injury and a myriad of individual unique characteristics, response can last days, week, or months.

Chronic inflammation, caused by scar tissue, autoimmune responses, infection, etc., can cause chronic algogenic pain .

3) Neuropathic Pain

This is pain that persists after all possible tissue healing has occurred. Once again, instant relief for this type of pain is not possible. This is chronic pain that may persist for months, years, or forever.

Lay people often view pain solely as a bad thing, but healthcare professionals recognize pain to be both friend and foe. For example, if one sits on one's foot for a prolonged period of time, it will eventually begin to hurt. This is an example of nociceptive pain. We simply self-diagnose and treat our foot pain by moving it or changing our sitting position, and the pain goes away.

People are constantly doing things that begin to generate pain, and the pain afferents send a sensory signal to our brain reminding us to stop doing that activity. In this regard, pain keeps us safe, reminding us not to do certain things or to stop doing certain things. Without pain, we would not survive childhood and make it into adulthood.

Chronic pain is another story.

Of the many structures that make up the spine, most of them are capable of generating pain. All of the spinal structures that can initiate the pain signal to the brain have a common factor: they are innervated by sensory afferent nociceptive neurons that carry the pain electrical signal to the brain. As noted by exceptional spine care pioneer Alf Acheson, MD, whatever causes spine pain must have a nerve (5). In 1991, Stephen Kuslich, MD, and colleagues clarified and quantified the spinal tissues that were capable of initiating the pain electrical signal to the brain as (6):

- Skin
- Superficial Muscles
- Deep Muscles
- Intervertebral Disc
- Facet Joint Capsules
- Periosteum of the Vertebral Bone
- Nerve roots

Any of these tissues are capable of initiating acute spinal pain. Chronic spinal pain perception was primarily attributed to the intervertebral disc and facet capsules, in that order (6). Other studies have primarily attributed chronic neck pain perception to the facet capsules and the intervertebral disc, in that reverse order (7).

For a new incidence of non-traumatic low back or neck pain, it is important for both clinicians and patients to make an initial quick assessment of the severity of the problem. Absent other historical indicators, it is common to assume the pain is algogenic in nature. This means there is an accumulation of algogenic inflammatory exudates that are increasing the sensitivity of the pain sensory nerves. The first step in doing this is to categorize the symptoms into one of three groups:

Group 1: Spinal pain alone

Either neck pain or back pain without pain radiation into the arms or legs. In general, algogenic spine pain that does not radiate is not serious. It is usually the consequence of a local inflammatory condition. It can be chronic and even disabling, but it is not dangerous.

Group 2: Sclerogenic pain; also known as sclerotomic pain or sclerotogenous pain

Sclerogenic pain radiates from the neck into the arm(s) or from the low back into the leg(s). Classically the pain radiation will not extend below the elbow (from the neck) or below the knee (from the low back).

As a rule, sclerogenic pain is difficult for the patient to localize. The pain presentation is often described as being deep and dull in character, similar to a toothache.

In general, sclerogenic pain is not dangerous. It is a form of referred pain that occurs as a consequence of a shared neuromere during embryonic development. In other words, the neurology of the back and the leg, or of the neck and the arm, are shared embryological, which can cause some confusion as to the exact location of the irritation when the electrical signal is sent to the brain. Originally based on the research of JH Kellgren and colleagues in 1938 and 1939, irritations of deep spinal tissues can cause sclerogenic pain referral to the arm or to the leg (8, 9).

In the sclerogenic pain patient, successful management of the deep spinal tissue irritations will resolve the sclerogenic pain referral. Deep spinal tissue irritations include irritations to the intervertebral disc, the facet joint capsules, and the core stabilization segmental mover muscles. These tissues respond excellently to spinal adjusting.

Group 3:   Radicular pain, radiculitis, and radiculopathy

The technical definition of radicular pain is that the spinal nerve root is inflamed, and the classic symptomatology is radiating arm or leg pain. In contrast to sclerogenic pain (a deep dull ache), the pain is often sharp and easily localized by the patient. Also, the pain often travels below the elbow (into the hands and fingers) and/or below the knee (into the foot and toes).

Radicular pain is more serious than sclerogenic pain. It is therefore a good idea to determine (to the best of one's ability) if the pain is radicular or sclerogenic . History and physical examination can be quite accurate in establishing a differential diagnosis. However, conformation will require advanced diagnostic imaging. The current gold standard in advanced diagnostic imaging is magnetic resonance imaging, or MRI.

Radicular pain is often caused by compression of the nerve root, the compression causing nerve root irritation and/or inflammation. This pathology is commonly referred to as compressive radiculopathy . Interestingly, the compression itself is not necessarily painful. Rather, the pain arises when the compression initiates irritation and/or inflammation of the nerve root. The degree of nerve root compression and its seriousness is estimated with MRI scans.

The most classic cause of radicular compression is herniation of the intervertebral disc. Other causes include arthritic changes (degenerative joint disease, degenerative disc disease, spondylosis) causing osseous (bone spurs, hypertrophic changes, osteophytes) narrowing of the intervertebral foramen.

Each nerve root supplies a specific patch of skin (a dermatome) and a specific muscle (a myotome). Consequently, radicular compression is often associated with specific myotomal muscle weakness and altered sensation in the dermatomal patch of skin (paresthesia).

The deep tendon reflex is a common component of establishing if the extremity pain is sclerogenic or radicular. With radicular compression , the deep tendon reflex is diminished or possibly even absent. There are three common deep tendon reflexes in the arms (assessing the nerve roots of the neck), and two in the legs (assessing the nerve roots in the low back).

Radicular compressive pathology can result in permanent death of some of the neurons in the nerve root, resulting in permanent loss of various functions. Consequently, when compressive radiculopathy is suspected, "red flags" of such pathology should be watched for and assessed. These "red flags" include:

- Progressive myotomal muscle weakness.
- Atrophy of the muscle.
- Saddle anesthesia (loss of sensation in the area of the buttocks that would contact a saddle when sitting).
- Loss of bowel, bladder, and/or sexual function.(difficulty starting, difficulty ending, dripping, loss of sensation, etc.)

There are two (one for the neck and one for the low back) very simple tests that are commonly done by healthcare providers to help determine if radiating pain is sclerogenic referral or as a consequence of radicular compression . These tests can also be easily performed by patients to help determine the seriousness of compression and its progress while under treatment.

Both tests are stretch tests. If the nerve root is compressed, irritated, and inflamed as it exits the spinal column, stretching it will aggravate the discomfort and the radiation.

Low Back Pain With Leg Radiation Test

This test is known as the Straight Leg Raising Test . It is also known as Laseque's Test , after Charles Laseque who first described the test in 1864 (10). The premise of the test is simple: movement of the leg causes movement of the lower lumbar nerve roots.

This test is performed by lying flat on one's back and raising one's leg up into the air while keeping the knee locked straight. Many normal people can do this to almost 90°. Individuals with lower back (lumbar) spinal radicular compression will begin to feel an increased in leg or back symptoms starting at about 35°.

According to Kapandji (11), when the leg is raised during the Straight Leg Raising Test , the lower lumbar spinal nerve roots will slide out of the nerve root hole (intervertebral foramen) by as much as half an inch (12 mm). If the nerve root is entrapped or compressed, the stretch will aggravate the irritation/inflammation, increasing symptoms.

It is accepted that the primary cause of compressive radiculopathy is herniation of the intervertebral disc. Most patients with discogenic compressive radiculopathy obtain symptomatic relief when lying down flat on their back. The probable explanation for this is that the intradiscal pressure is least when in this position (12, 13)

In contrast, it is established that when one sits down, intradiscal pressures are increased by roughly a factor of 6 (25 psi to 140 psi) (12, 13).

Therefore it is argued that performing the Straight Leg Raising Test when sitting down is a better indicator of the presence of discogenic compressive radiculopathy . This test is known as Bechterew's Test. It is performed by sitting up straight, and then straightening out one's leg until it is parallel with the horizon. An increase in leg or spinal symptomatology is considered to be a positive indicator of the presence of low back/leg compressive radiculopathy.

Brachial Plexus Tension Test of Elvey

The test that is an equivalent to the lower back Straight Leg Raising Test in the neck (cervical spine) is the Brachial Plexus Tension Test of Elvey . This test was originally described by Australian physiotherapist Robert Elvey in 1986 (14). Once again, the premise of the test is simple: movement of the arm causes movement of the lower cervical spine nerve roots.

The step-by-step procedure for performing the Brachial Plexus Tension Test of Elvey are well described by Quintner in the British Journal of Rheumatology in 1989 (15):

TO START:

Put the patient supine.

Externally rotate the arm and supinate the forearm.

Flex the fingers, wrist, and elbow.

Abduct the shoulder joint 110 degrees, so that the elbow is superior to the glenohumeral joint.

Put the arm behind the coronal plane of the body.

TO ASSESS:

Keep the shoulder girdle depressed.

Keep the forearm supinated.

Extend the elbow.

Extend the wrist, supination of the forearm.

Extend the fingers.

IF NEGATIVE:

Reassess with the head/neck laterally flexed to the opposite side.

Summary

Both cervical spine and lumbar spine compressive radiculopathies are coupled with a worse prognosis for complete recovery. Compressive radiculopathy typically requires more frequent treatment and more prolonged treatment. Compressive radiculopathy patients often have more long-term subjective and objective residuals, and more disability. Patients with compressive radiculopathy often require advanced imaging (such as MRI) for a full assessment of their pathology. Occasionally, patients with compressive radiculopathy will require a surgical decompression. These patients should always be monitored for the emergence of "red flag" signs.

The Straight Leg Raising Test (Laseque's) and the Brachial Plexus Tension Test (Elvey) are simple tests to assess the presence of a compressive radiculopathic process.

Low Back Pain – What To Do Immediately (Part 1)

This article is part 1 of a 2 part series. For Part 2, **click here**.

Low back pain (LBP) will most likely strike at some point for all of us, at least that's what statistically happens. How we "deal with it" initially can be critical in its progression or cessation. Here are some "highlights" of what to do "WHEN" this happens to you.

STOP: The most important thing you can do is STOP what you are doing. That is, IF you're "lucky enough" to be pre-warned BEFORE the crisis point of LBP strikes. This step can be critical, as once it hurts "too much," it may be too late to quickly reverse the process. The "cause" of LBP is often cumulative, meaning it occurs gradually over time, usually from repetitive motion that overloads the region. As stated previously, "IF YOU'RE LUCKY" you'll be warned BEFORE LBP becomes a disabling/preventing activity. Typically, when the tissues in the low back are over-stressed and initially injured, the nerve endings in the injured tissue trigger muscle guarding as a protective mechanism. This reflex "muscle spasm" restricts blood flow resulting in more pain creating a vicious cycle that needs to be STOPPED!

REACT: This is the "hard part" as it requires you to perform something specifically, but once you prove to yourself that this approach really works, you won't hesitate. You'll need to determine your "direction preference", or the position that reduces LBP. Once established, you can perform exercises to help mitigate your back pain. To make this work, you must be able to perform these exercises in public without drawing too much attention so you can feel comfortable doing them at any time at any place.

EXERCISE A: If BENDING FORWARD feels relieving, the exercise of choice is to sit and a) cross one leg over the other, b) pull that knee towards the opposite shoulder, and c) move the knee in various positions so the area of "pull" changes. Work out each tight area by adding an arch to the low back, rotate your trunk towards the side of the flexed knee (sit up tall and twist – if it doesn't hurt) and alternate between these positions (10-15 seconds at a time) until the stretched area feels "loosened up." A second exercise is to sit and rotate the trunk until a stretch is felt. Again, alternate between different degrees of low back arching during the twists, feeling for different areas of stretch until it feels looser, usually 5-15 seconds per side. A third exercise is to sit and bend forward, as if to tie a shoe, and hold that position until the tightness "melts away."

EXERCISE B: If BENDING BACKWARDS feels best, exercise options include placing your fists in the small of your back and leaning backwards over the fists, or bending backward and holding the position as long as needed to feel relief (usually 5-15 seconds). From a sitting position, try placing a rolled-up towel (make one with a towel rolled tightly like a sleeping bag held with rubber bands) in the small of the back to increase the curve. Lying on your back with the roll and a pillow under the low back can also feel great!

Low Back Pain – What To Do Immediately (Part 2)

Low back pain (LBP), as previously stated, will affect most (if not all) of us at some point in time. Knowing what to do when the warning signs occur is essential to avoiding a disabling level of LBP. Last month, we started the discussion about offering ways to manage the LBP using exercises with the objective of stopping and reversing a potentially serious level of LBP. We offered ways of stretching from a sitting position that can be done in public. Here are some standing exercise options.

1. EXERCISE C: THE HAMSTRING & GROIN STRETCH: From standing 1) Place your foot up onto a seat, bench, chair, pipe of a railing, or anything about knee level (it doesn't have to be very high). If your balance isn't very good, make sure to hold onto a wall or counter to keep your balance. 2) Keep your knee bent 20-30 degrees and arch your lower back by sticking out the buttocks until you feel the pull or stretch in the hamstrings (back of the leg). 3) Slowly straighten your knee (keep the buttocks poked out and the low back arched) and you will feel the hamstrings gradually get tighter. 4) Change the angle of the knee and/or the amount of l ow back arch/pelvic tilt to modify the pulling intensity in the hamstrings. Continue this stretch for 15-30 seconds or until you feel the muscles loosening up. 5) Stay in that EXACT SAME POSITION and rotate your torso inwards (towards the leg you're standing on) until you will feel the pull change from the hamstrings to the groin (inside thigh) muscles. You can also go back and forth between the hamstrings and the groin (adductor) muscles and continue the exercise until the back of the leg

and groin feel adequately stretched (usually 5 to 15 seconds/leg).

2. EXERCISE D: THE HIP FLEXOR STRETCH: From standing: 1) Step forwards with one leg and stand in a semi-long, stride position (one foot ahead of the other). 2) On the back leg side, rotate the pelvis forwards until the hip lines up with the forward leg hip (or, the pelvis is square). 3) Add a posterior pelvic tilt (tuck in your buttock/pelvis or, flatten your low back). 4) Lean backwards (extend the low back) holding the above position. As you extend back, feel for the pull deep inside the upper front part of the thigh/groin area. You can alter between the third and fourth steps to release and re-stretch the hip flexor. Continue the stretch for 5-15 seconds or until you feel it's stretched out and repeat on the opposite side. This one takes a little work but once you feel it, you will see why it's so good!

3. EXERCISE E: THE ADDUCTOR STRETCH: As an alternative to the second part of EXERCISE C (step 5 of the standing hamstring stretch), stand with your legs spread apart fairly wide. Shift your pelvis from side to side (left then right) and feel for the stretch on the inner thigh/groin region. You can increase the stretch by adding a lean to the side you're shifting the pelvis. Try holding the stretch for 5-15 seconds, alternating between sides 5-10 times.

These exercises are meant to be done in public WHEN you need to stretch. Stop the vicious cycle from getting out of control by STOPPING, STRETCHING, and then resuming your activity if you can!

The Mysteries of Low Back Pain!

Do you realize how complicated the low back region is when it comes to investigating the cause of low back pain (LBP)? There can be findings on an x-ray, MRI, or CT scan such as degenerative disk disease, arthritis, even bulging and/or herniated disks that have NOTHING to do with why the back hurts. Similarly, there are often other abnormal findings present in many of us who have NO low back pain whatsoever! Because of this seemingly paradoxical situation, we as clinicians must be careful not to over-diagnose based on the presence of these "abnormal findings" AND on the same hand, be careful not to under-diagnose them as well.

Looking further into this interesting paradox, one study reported findings that support this point. Investigators examined 67 asymptomatic individuals who had NO prior history of low back pain and evaluated them using magnetic resonant imaging (MRI). They found 21 of the 67 (31%) had an identifiable disk and/or spinal canal abnormality (which is where the spinal cord and nerves run). Seven years later, this same group of non-suffering individuals were once again contacted to see if they had developed any back problems within that time frame. The goal of the study was to determine if one could "predict" who might develop low back pain based on certain abnormal imaging findings in non-suffering subjects. A questionnaire was sent to each of these individuals, of which 50 completed and returned the questionnaire. A repeat MRI scan was performed on 31 of these subjects, and two neurologists and one orthopedic spine surgeon interpreted the MRI studies using a blinded approach (without having knowledge about the subject's symptoms or lack thereof). Each level was assessed for abnormalities including disk bulging/herniation and degeneration. Those who had initial abnormal findings were defined as "progressed" (worsened) if an increased severity of the original finding was evident or if additional or new spinal levels had become involved over the seven-year time span.

Of the 50 who returned the questionnaire, 29 (58%) had NO low back pain, while 21 had developed LBP. In the original group that had the MRI repeated seven years later, new MRI findings included the following: twelve remained "normal," five had herniated disks, three had developed spinal stenosis, and one had "moderate" disk degeneration. Regarding radiating leg pain, four of the eight had abnormal findings originally, two of the eight had spinal stenosis, one had a disk protrusion, and one an "extruded" ("ruptured") disk. In general, repeat MRI scans revealed a greater frequency of disk herniation, bulging, degeneration, and spinal stenosis compared to the original scans. Those with the longest duration of LBP did NOT have the greatest degree of abnormalities on the original scans. They concluded that the original MRI findings were NOT PREDICTIVE of future development of LBP.

They summarized, "…clinical correlation is essential to determine the importance of abnormalities on MR images." These findings correlate well with other studies, such as 50% or more of all asymptomatic people HAVE bulging disks and approximately 30% of us have herniated disks – WITHOUT PAIN. To be of diagnostic (clinical) value, the person MUST have signs and symptoms that agree with the imaging test, which is used to CONFIRM the diagnosis. Bottom line, If you have LBP, come see us, as we will evaluate and treat YOU, NOT your x-rays (or MRI) findings!

I Slipped a Disk – What Is That Exactly?

"I was digging a hole in my garden and hit a rock with the shovel. After clearing the dirt from around the rock, I bent over and reached into the hole. I couldn't get a good grip on the rock and had to twist my body to get my arm under it. As I started to move the rock, I felt something 'give out' in my lower back and felt immediate low back pain, but it wasn't terrible. Like a fool, I gave it another try but this time, the **pain in my back** was really sharp when I twisted to reach under it. Then, it felt like a knife stabbing me when I tried to stand up. Since then, I can't stand up straight and pain is shooting down my left leg."

The intervertebral disk is like a shock-absorber located between each vertebra in our spine extending from the tail bone to the upper neck. When healthy, your disks truly do function as shock absorbers. There are two parts to the disk – the inner part (called the nucleus) which is the liquid-like center and the tough, laminated, and rubber-like outer part (the annulus) that hold the nucleus in the center of the disk. The annulus has concentric rings which look similar to the rings of an oak tree trunk and the strength of these laminated rings is due to the fibers crisscrossing, creating a self-sealing, secure border for the nucleus center. In spite of this great anatomical structure, our disks degenerate and can crack or tear allowing the more liquid-like nucleus to leak out of the annulus creating the classic "slipped disk" (technically referred to as a herniated or ruptured disk). When the herniated disk presses into the nerve that goes down the leg, pain is felt along its course and can radiate all the way to the foot. There are five vertebrae and disks with a pair of nerves that go into each leg and depending which disk ruptures, pain will follow a different course down the leg. This is why your chiropractor may ask you if you feel the pain more in the back or in the front of the leg. When the disk tears prior to both disk herniation and leg pain, low back pain occurs because the nerve fibers that are normally only located in the outer third of the disk grow into the central portion of the disk, causing it to generate more pain.

So, now for the important question, "…what can I do for it?" When you visit a doctor of chiropractic, her or she will ask you about how you injured your back. Often, the cause of a herniated disk can be the accumulation of multiple events over time. It certainly can happen after one major event, like our example of lifting a rock out of a hole, but that is usually the "straw that breaks the camel's back" and not the sole cause. Many researchers report it is rare for a healthy disk to herniate. Rather, disk degeneration with tears already present sets up the situation where a bend plus a twist, "…finishes the job." An orthopedic and neurological examination will usually clearly identify the level of herniation. Chiropractic treatment often includes traction types of techniques, some form of spinal manipulation or mobilization, extension exercises, and physical therapy modalities like electric stimulation, low level laser, or ultrasound, and ice therapy. Core / trunk strengthening and posture management are also

Commonly applied and proper lifting/pulling/pushing techniques are taught.

Back Pain Study Shows Great Results For This Treatment

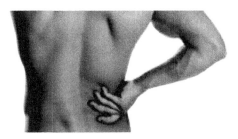

Lacey / Olympia – Science is amazing. The pace that new treatments are developed with cutting-edge technology is mind boggling.

What is just as incredible is how sometimes research chows old treatments research shows old treatments are much more effective than once thought.

For example, a 2014 study published in *Journal of Manipulative and Physiological Therapeutics* said this about a back pain treatment that is at least 120 years old: "The proportion of patients reporting clinically relevant improvement in this current study is surprisingly good, with nearly 70% of patients improved as early as 2 weeks after the start of their treatment. By 3 months, this figure was up to 90.5% and then stabilized at 6 months and 1 year."

What's the treatment?

The treatment is spinal manipulative therapy – and if you have back pain – you should know what else this study said...

"This study shows that patients with proven lumbar intervertebral disc herniation and compressive neuropathology that receive traditional chiropractic side posture manipulation is both safe and effective. The ultimate clinical effectiveness of about 90% is impressive when compared to any form of therapy, and with no reported serious side effects.

This study would suggest that all patients suffering from lumbar intervertebral disc herniation with compressive neuropathology should be treated with chiropractic spinal adjusting."

Who Should Try This Treatment?

You are a good candidate for this treatment if you have: (1) Acute low back pain with or without leg pain, (2) low back pain with herniated or bulging disc – with or without leg pain. (3) chronic low back pain.

It is important to note that no one should expect the results from this study or any other study. All patients are different and all cases are individual.

That's why it is important to be evaluated by a qualified physician to see if this treatment is right for you.

For that reason, Dr. David Warwick is offering complimentary consultations to back pain sufferers. If you would like a consultation, just call **360-951-4504**. There is no cost or obligation and you will get your questions answered and find out if this treatment can help you. **Contact** Dr. David Warwick today!

Low Back Manipulation
How Does it Work?

Low **back pain** (LBP) is such a common problem that if you haven't suffered from it yet, you probably will eventually. Here are a few facts to consider: 1) LBP affects men and women equally; 2) It is most common between ages 30-50; 3) Sedentary (non-active) lifestyles contribute a lot to causation; 4) Too much or too little exercise can result in LBP; 5) A BMI around 25 is "ideal" for weight management, which helps prevent LBP; 6) Causes of LBP include lifestyle (activity level), genetics – including, but not limited to, weight and osteoarthritis; 7) Occupation; 8) Exercise habits, and the list can go on and on. Let's next look at how an adjustment is done.
When spinal manipulation is performed in the low-back region, the patient is often placed in a side lying position with the upper leg flexed towards the chest and the bottom leg kept straight. The bottom shoulder is pulled forwards and the upper shoulder is rotated backwards at the same time the low back area receives that the manipulation is rotated forwards. This produces a twisting type of motion that is well within the normal range of joint motion. When the adjustment is made, a "high velocity" (or quick), "low amplitude" (a short distance of movement) thrust is delivered often resulting in "cavitation" (the crack or, release of gases). So, WHY do we do this?

Most studies show that when there is back pain, there is inflammation. In fact, inflammation is found in most disease processes that occur both within and outside the musculoskeletal system. We know that when we control inflammation, pain usually subsides. That is why the use of "PRICE" (Protect, Rest, Ice, Compress, Elevate) works well for most muscle/joint painful conditions. We have also learned that IF we can avoid cortisone and non-steroidal drugs (like aspirin, ibuprofen, naproxen, etc.), tissues heal quicker and better, so these SHOULD BE AVOIDED ! If you didn't know that, check out:

http://www.benthamscience.com/open/torehj/articles/V 006/1TOREHJ.pdf

Please see our prior discussions on the use of anti-inflammatory herbs and diets that are MUCH safer than non-steroidal drugs! But what does spinal manipulation DO in reference to inflammation?

Different things occur physiologically during a spinal adjustment or manipulation. We know that the mechanical receptors located in muscles, muscle tendons, ligaments, and joint capsules are stimulated and this results in muscle relaxation (reduced spasm or tightness), increased measurable range of motion, and a decrease in pain. A recent study also reported that inflammatory markers (CRP and interleukin-6) measured in a blood test, NORMALIZED after a series of nine chiropractic low back manipulations! So, NOT ONLY do spinal adjustments give immediate improvements in pain, flexibility, and muscle relaxation, they also REDUCE INFLAMMATION without the use of any pharmaceuticals!

So, let's review what manipulation does for your low back pain: 1) Pain reduction; 2) Improved flexibility – now you can put on your socks with less pain and strain; 3) Improved functions and activities of daily living like sitting more comfortably, getting in or out of your car, bending over to feed the cat, etc.; 4) Improved sleep quality; and 5) Faster healing time by actually reducing the inflammatory markers in the blood! If you have LBP, PLEASE don't delay – make that appointment TODAY!

Can Chiropractic Help the Post-Surgical Patient?

Low **back pain** (LBP) accounts for over 3 million emergency department visits per year in the United States alone. Worldwide, LBP affects approximately 84% of the general population, so eventually almost EVERYONE will have lower back pain that requires treatment! There is evidence dating back to the early Roman and Greek era that indicates back pain was also very prevalent, and that really hasn't changed. Some feel it's because we are bipedal (walk on two legs) rather than quadrupedal (walk on four limbs). When comparing the two, degenerative disk disease and spinal osteoarthritis are postponed in the four-legged species by approximately two (equivalent) decades. But regardless of the reason, back pain is "the rule," NOT the exception when it comes to patient visits to chiropractors and medical doctors. Previously, we looked at the surgical rate of low back pain by comparing patients who initially went to spinal surgeons vs. to chiropractors, and we were amazed! Remember? Approximately 43% of workers who first saw a surgeon had surgery compared to ONLY 1.5% of those who first saw a chiropractor! So, the questions this month are, how successful IS spinal surgery, and what about all those patients who have had surgery but still have problems – can chiropractic still help them?

A review of the literature published in the Journal of the American Academy of Orthopedic Surgeons showed that in most cases of degenerative disk disease (DDD), non-surgical approaches are the most effective treatment choice (that includes chiropractic!). They report the success rate of spinal fusions for DDD has been only 50-60%. The advent of artificial disks, which originally proposed to be a "cure" for symptomatic disk disease, has fared no better with possible worse long-term problems that are not yet fully understood. They state, "Surgery should be the last option, but too often patients think of surgery as a cure-all and are eager to embark on it." They go on to write, "Also, surgeons should pay close attention to the list of contraindications, and recommend surgery only for those patients who are truly likely to benefit from it." Another study reported that, when followed for 10 years after artificial disk surgery, a similar 40% of the patients treated failed and had a second surgery within three years after the first! Similar findings are reported for post-surgical spinal stenosis as well as other spinal conditions.

So what about the success rate of chiropractic management for patients who have had low back surgery? In a 2012 article, three patients who had prior lumbar spinal fusions at least two years previous were treated with spinal manipulation (three treatments over three consecutive days) followed by rehabilitation for eight weeks. At the completion of care, all three (100%) had clinical improvement that were still maintained a year later. Another study reported 32 cases of post-surgical low back pain patients undergoing chiropractic care resulted in an average drop in pain from 6.4/10 to 2.3/10 (that means pain was reduced by 4.1 points out of 10 or, 64%). An even larger drop was reported when dividing up those who had a combination of spinal surgeries (discectomy, fusion, and/or laminectomy) with a pain drop of 5.7 out of 10 points!

Typically, spinal surgery SHOULD be the last resort, but we now know that is not always practiced. IF a patient has had more than one surgery and still has pain, the term "failed back syndrome" is applied and carries many symptoms and disability. Again, to NOT utilize chiropractic post-surgically seems almost as foolish as not utilizing it pre-surgically! GIVE US A CALL!!!

Low Back Pain: Surgery vs. Chiropractic?

Low **back pain** (LBP) is the second most common cause of disability in the United States (US) and a very common reason for lost days at work with an estimated 149 million days of work lost per year. The total cost associated with this is astronomical at between $100-200 billion/yr., of which 2/3rds are due to decreased wages and productivity. More than 80% of the population will have an episode of LBP at some point in their lifetime. The good news is that 95% recover within two to three months of onset. However, some never recover which leads to chronic LBP (LBP > 3 months), and 20-44% will have a recurrence of LBP within one year with lifetime recurrences of up to 85%! What this means is that most of us have, have had, or will have LBP, and we'll get it again! So the question is, what are we going to do about it?

Surgery has traditionally been considered a "last resort" with less invasive approaches recommended first. Chiropractic adjustments and management strategies have traditionally faired very well when compared to other non-surgical methods like physical therapy, acupuncture, and massage therapy. But, is there evidence that by receiving chiropractic treatment, low back surgery can be avoided? Let's take a look!

A recent study was designed to determine whether or not we could predict those who would require low back surgery within three years of a job-related back injury. This is a very important study as back injuries are the most common occupational injury in the US, and few studies have investigated what, if any, early predictors of future spine surgery after work-related injury exist. The study reviewed cases of 1,885 Washington state workers, of which 174 or 9.2% had low back surgery within three years. The initial predictors of surgery included high disability scores on questionnaires, greater injury severity, and seeing a surgeon as the first provider after the injury. Reduced odds of having surgery included: 1)

If this isn't enough evidence, another recent study (University of British Columbia) looked at the safety of spine surgery and reported that (taken from a group of 942 LBP surgical patients): 1) 87% had at least one documented complication; 2) 39% of the 87% had to stay longer in the hospital as a result; 3) 10.5% had a complication during the surgery; 4) 73.5% had a post-surgical complication (which included: 8% delirium, 7% pneumonia, 5% nerve pain, 4.5% had difficulty swallowing, 3% nerve deterioration, 13.5% wound complication); 5) 14 people died as a surgical complication. Another study showed lower annual healthcare costs for those receiving chiropractic vs. those who did not. The "take-home" message is clear: TRY CHIROPRACTIC FIRST!!!

Low Back Pain – Is it on the Rise?

As stated last month, the prevalence of low **back pain** (LBP) is REALLY high! In fact, it's the second most common cause of disability among adults in the United States (US) and a very common reason for lost days at work. The total cost of back pain in the US, including treatment and lost productivity, ranges between $100 billion to $200 billion a year! Is low back pain on the rise, staying the same, or lessening? Let's take a look!

In the past two decades, the use of health care services for chronic LBP (that means LBP > 3 months) has substantially increased. When reviewing studies reporting insurance claims information, researchers note a significant increase in the use of spinal injections, surgery, and narcotic prescriptions. There has been an increase in the use of spinal manipulation by chiropractors as well, along with increased physical therapy services and primary care physician driven non-narcotic prescriptions. In general, LBP sufferers who are chronic (vs. acute) are the group using most of these services and incurring the majority of costs. The reported utilization of the above mentioned services was only 3.9% in 1992 compared to 10.2% in 2006, just 11 years later. The question now becomes, why is this? Possible reasons for this increase health care use in chronic LBP sufferers may be: 1) There are simply more people suffering from chronic LBP; 2) More chronic LBP patients are deciding to seek care or treatment where previously they "just accepted and lived with it" and didn't pursue treatment; or, 3) A combination of these factors. Regardless of which of the above three is most accurate, the most important issue is, what can we do to help chronic back pain sufferers?

As we've discussed in the past, an anti-inflammatory diet, exercise within YOUR personal tolerance level, not smoking, getting enough sleep, and obtaining chiropractic adjustments every two weeks are well documented methods of "controlling" chronic LBP (as there really ISN'T a "cure" in many cases). You may be surprised to hear that maintenance care has good literature support for controlling chronic LBP. In the 8/15/11 issue of SPINE (Vol. 36, No. 18, pp1427-1437), two Medical Doctors (MDs) penned the article, "Does Maintained Spinal Manipulation Therapy for Chronic Nonspecific Low Back Pain Result in Better Long-Term Outcomes?" Here, they took 60 patients with chronic LBP (cLBP) and randomly assigned them into one of three groups: 1) 12 treatments of sham (fake) SMT (spinal manipulation) have over a one month period; 2) 12 treatments, over a one month period but no treatment for the following nine months; or 3) 12 treatments for one month AND then SMT every two weeks for the following nine months. To measure the differences between the three groups, they measured pain, disability, generic health status, and back-specific patient satisfaction at baseline, 1-, 4-, 7-, and 10-month time intervals. They found only the patients in the second and third groups experienced significantly lower pain and disability scores vs. the first group after the first month of treatments (at three times a week). BUT, only the third group showed more improvement at the 10-month evaluation. Also, by the tenth month, the pain and disability scores returned back to nearly the initial baseline/initial level in group two. The authors concluded that, "To obtain long-term benefit, this study suggests maintenance SM after the initial intensive manipulative therapy." Other studies have reported fewer medical tests, lower costs, fewer doctor visits, less work absenteeism, and a higher quality of life when maintenance chiropractic visits are utilized. The question is, WHEN will insurance companies and general practitioners start RECOMMENDING chiropractic maintenance care for chronic LBP patients?

Low Back Pain and Balance Specific Exercises

Low **back pain** (LBP) and its relationship to balance has been the topic for the past two Health Updates, and an initial discussion regarding specific balance exercises was introduced last month. This month's Health Update will complete the discussion about what you can do to preserve your current balance skills, or better yet, improve them! Remember, wear your foot orthotics and don't forget to move them between your different shoes. Similarly, if you have leg length imbalance, move your heel lift to other shoes or simply purchase additional lifts and keep the heel lift in several pairs of shoes. Also, test your balance skills now before starting a balance exercise program and re-test every 2-4 weeks to measure improvement (see the January 2013 Health Update for the testing protocol).

The initial exercise we discussed was standing with your feet together and holding that position for progressively longer times (eyes open and closed). Once you can hold this position with your eyes closed for = 30 seconds, start increasing the balance challenge by:

1. Move your heel of the left foot next to the big toe of the right foot and repeat the exercise with the eyes open and closed. Repeat on the other side! When successful for =30 sec., do it with eyes closed.....
2. Place your left foot in front of the right foot/toes (like standing on a balance beam) and repeat the exercise with the eyes open and closed. Repeat on the other side! When successful for =30 sec., do it with eyes closed.....
3. Repeat #1 and #2 standing on a thin pillow and/or a wobble cushion or rocker board, making sure you are "safe" by standing in the corner of a room or in an entrance to a room where you can grab the door frame when needed. DO NOT RISK falling!
4. Rocker board exercise options:

- Rock forwards/backwards (FW/BW) looking straight ahead (don't look down at your feet). Make sure the board you are using is "safe" (where you can safely step off forwards and backwards). Don't use a board that is too high off the ground (about 3" is

maximum). Repeat the FW/BW rocking slowly for 10 minutes periodically opening and closing your eyes.
- Repeat "A" but stand at a 45° angle to the front/back direction so you are rocking at an angle using the same methods and time frame.
- Repeat "A" but stand at a 90° angle to the front/back direction so you are rocking at an angle using a similar method and time frame.

You can then "make up" exercises standing on the rocker board or cushion like simulating a golf swing, tennis stroke, or other favorite sport, yoga move, etc. Be creative and make it fun!!!

Where Exactly Does Back Pain Come From?

In this month's edition we're going to discuss some "intrigue" that has plagued low back treatments both conservative and aggressive for many years now.

The intrigue being "WHERE" exactly does the pain generate from. What structure? What neurological mechanism? And with some detective work I think we've uncovered some significant findings.

The modern era in the understanding of low back pain that we're in right now began in 1976 when internationally respected orthopedic surgeon Alf Nachemson published his detailed review (136 references) in the new journal SPINE (1), entitled "The Lumbar Spine: An Orthopedic Challenge ".

In this article, Dr. Nachemson notes that a staggering 80% of us will experience low **back pain** at some time in our life. He further notes that:

"The Intervertebral Disc Is Most Likely The Cause Of The Pain…"

Dr. Nachemson makes a VERY convincing case when he presents 6 lines of reasoning, supported by 17 references, to support his contention that the intervertebral disc is the most likely source of back pain, including the primary research completed by Smyth and Wright in 1958 (2). Regarding the work by Smyth and Wright, Dr. Nachemson notes:

"Investigations have been performed in which thin nylon threads were surgically fastened to various structures and around the nerve root. Three to four weeks after surgery these structures were irritated by pulling on the threads, but pain resembling that which the patient had experienced previously could only be registered only from the outer part of the annulus" of the disc.

It had been established in the 1930s that herniation of the lumbar disc could put pressure on the nerve root or the cauda equine, resulting in sciatica. However, Dr. Nachemson in this context is saying something dramatically different;

He's Claiming That A Non-Herniated Disc Problem Was Causing Back Pain.

At the time (1976), claiming the intervertebral disc was capable of initiating pain was new and not only that, Nachemson claiming the disc to be the most probable source of back pain was both surprising AND revolutionary.

At the time, most authoritative reference texts stated the intervertebral disc was not even innervated with pain afferents and therefore not capable of initiating pain.

As an example, rheumatology professor Malcolm Jayson, MD (editor) in the 1987 text titled The Lumbar Spine and Back Pain , states

"in the mature human spine no nerve endings of any description remain in the nucleus pulposus or annulus fibrosis of the intervertebral disc in any region of the vertebral column." (3)

A conclusion we now know to be 100% false.

Support for Dr. Nachemson's contention of disc pain came in 1981 when anatomist and physician Nikoli Bogduk published an extensive review of the literature on the topic of disc innervation, along with his own primary research, in the prestigious Journal of Anatomy (4). Dr. Bogduk notes:

"In the absence of any comprehensive description of the innervation of the lumbar intervertebral discs and their related longitudinal ligaments, the present study was undertaken to establish in detail the source and pattern of innervation of these structures."

Dr. Bogduk and his team concluded decisively:

"The Lumbar Intervertebral Discs Are Supplied By A Variety Of Nerves."
and "Clinically, The Concept Of 'Disc Pain' Is Now Well Accepted."

Dr. Bogduk returned in 1983 updating his research notes in SPINE, stating more specifically :

"THE LUMBAR INTERVERTEBRAL DISCS ARE INNERVATED

posteriorly by the sinuvertebral nerves, but laterally by

branches of the ventral rami and grey rami communicantes...

The posterior longitudinal ligament is innervated by the sinuvertebral nerves and the anterior longitudinal ligament by branches of the grey rami.

Lateral and intermediate branches of the lumbar dorsal rami supply the iliocostalis lumborum and longissimus thoracis, respectively.

Medial branches supply the multifidus, intertransversarii mediales, interspinales, interspinous ligament, and the lumbar zygapophysial joints."

"The distribution of the intrinsic nerves of the lumbar vertebral column

systematically identifies those structures that are

potential sources of primary low-back pain ."

Adding to the growing momentum of this "disc-pain" concept... In 1987, SPINE published Dr. Vert Mooney's Presidential Address of the International Society for the Study of the Lumbar Spine. It was delivered at the 13th Annual Meeting of the International Society for the Study of the Lumbar Spine, May 29-June 2, 1986, Dallas, Texas, and titled (6):

Where Is the Pain Coming From?

In this article, Dr. Mooney notes the following:

"Six weeks to 2 months is usually enough to heal any stretched ligament, muscle tendon, or joint capsule.

Yet we know that 10% of back 'injuries' do not resolve in 2 months and that they do become chronic."

"Anatomically the motion segment of the back is made up of two synovial joints and a unique relatively avascular tissue found nowhere else in the body – the intervertebral disc. Is it possible for the disc to obey different rules of damage than the rest of the connective tissue of the musculoskeletal system?"

"Persistent pain in the back with referred pain to the leg is largely on the basis of abnormalities within the disc."

Chemistry of the disc is based on the relationship between mucopolysaccharide production and water content.

"Mechanical events can be translated into chemical events related to pain."

An important aspect of disc nutrition and health is the mechanical aspects of the disc related to the fluid mechanics.

"Mechanical activity has a great deal to do with the exchange of water and oxygen concentration" in the disc.

The pumping action maintains the nutrition and biomechanical function of the intervertebral disc. Thus, "research substantiates the view that unchanging posture, as a result of constant pressure such as standing, sitting or lying, leads to an interruption of pressure-dependent transfer of liquid. Actually the human intervertebral disc lives because of movement."

"The fluid content of the disc can be changed by mechanical activity, and the fluid content is largely bound to the proteoglycans, especially of the nucleus."

"In summary, what is the answer to the question of where is the pain coming from in the chronic low-back pain patient? I believe its source, ultimately, is in the disc. Basic studies and clinical experience suggest that mechanical therapy is the most rational approach to relief of this painful condition."

"Prolonged rest and passive physical therapy modalities no longer have a place in the treatment of the chronic problem."

This model presented by Dr. Mooney in this paper goes on to discuss:

The intervertebral disc as the primary source of both back pain and referred leg pain. The disc apparently becomes painful because of altered biochemistry, which sensitizes the pain afferents that innervate it.

Disc biochemistry is altered because of mechanical problems , especially mechanical problems that reduce disc movement.

Therefore, the most rational approach to the treatment of chronic low back pain is mechanical therapy that restores the motion to the joints of the spine, especially to the disc.

Prolonged Rest Is Inappropriate Management

Additional support for the disc being the primary source of back pain was presented by Dr. Stephen Kuslich in the prestigious journal Orthopedic Clinics of North America in April 1991 (7). The title of his article is:

The Tissue Origin of Low Back Pain and Sciatica:
A Report of Pain Response to Tissue Stimulation During Operations
on the Lumbar Spine Using Local Anesthesia

These authors performed 700 lumbar spine operations using only local anesthesia to determine the tissue origin of low back and leg pain, and they present the results on 193 consecutive patients studied prospectively. Several of their critically important findings for you include:

"Back pain could be produced by several lumbar tissues, but by far, the most common tissue or origin was the outer layer of the annulus fibrosis."

The lumbar fascia could be "touched or even cut without anesthesia."

Any pain derived from muscle pressure was "derived from local vessels and nerves, rather than the muscle bundles themselves."

"The normal, uncompressed, or unstretched nerve root was completely insensitive to pain."

"In spite of all that has been written about muscles, fascia, and bone as a source of pain, these tissues are really quite insensitive."

In summary, these authors found that...The Outer Annulus Is "THE SITE" Of A Patient's Back Pain.

Past studies that suggest the disc is not an important source of low back pain because nerve endings "are not present" are clearly and overwhelmingly erroneous when you carefully analyzed the most modern literature.

Documented research at no time has demonstrated irritation of a normal or inflamed nerve root to produce low back pain. Back muscles themselves are proven not to be a source of back pain; in fact, the muscles, fascia, and bone are really quite insensitive for pain. The inflamed, stretched, or compressed nerve root is in fact the cause of buttock, leg pain and sciatica, but not back pain.

Very recently in 2006, physician researchers from Japan published in SPINE the results of an extremely sophisticated immunohistochemistry study of the sensory innervation of the human lumbar intervertebral disc (8). The article is titled: The Degenerated Lumbar Intervertebral Disc is Innervated Primarily by Peptide-Containing Sensory Nerve Fibers in Humans

The Japanese researchers note: "Many investigators have reported the existence of sensory nerve fibers in the intervertebral discs of animals and humans, suggesting that the intervertebral disc can be a source of low back pain."

"Both inner and outer layers of the degenerated lumbar intervertebral disc are innervated by pain sensory nerve fibers in humans."

Pain neuron fibers are found in all human discs that have been removed because they are the source of a patient's chronic low back pain.

The nerve fibers in the disc, found in this study, "indicates that the disc can be a source of pain sensation."

The information and data offered by these studies from across 30 years of published research in the most highly respected journals CLEARLY and UNEQUIVOCALLY demonstrates that...

The Annulus Of The Intervertebral Disc Is Primarily Responsible For The Majority Of Chronic Low Back Pain.

Above (6), Dr. Vert Mooney notes in his Presidential Address to the International Society for the Study of the Lumbar Spine that, "basic studies and clinical experience suggest that mechanical therapy is the most rational approach to relief of this painful [intervertebral disc] condition."

In Support Of Dr. Mooney's Perspective, Four Such Studies Are Reviewed Here: In 1985, Dr. Kirkaldy-Willis, a Professor Emeritus of Orthopedics and director of the Low-Back Pain Clinic at the University Hospital, Saskatoon, Canada, published an article in the journal Canadian Family Physician (9).

In this study, the authors present the results of a prospective observational study of spinal manipulation in 283 patients with chronic low back and leg pain.

All 283 patients in this study had failed prior conservative and/or operative treatment, and they were all totally disabled. These patients were given a "two or three week regimen of daily spinal manipulations by an experienced chiropractor."

These authors determined a good result from manipulation to be: "Symptom-free with no restrictions for work or other activities."

OR

"Mild intermittent pain with no restrictions for work or other activities."

81% of the patients with referred pain syndromes subsequent to joint dysfunctions achieved the "good" result.

48% of the patients with nerve compression syndromes, primarily subsequent to disc lesions and/or central canal spinal stenosis, achieved the "good" result.

Dr. Kirkaldy-Willis attributed this clinical outcome to Melzack and Wall's 1965 "Gate Theory of Pain." He noted that the manipulation improved motion, which improved proprioceptive neurological input into the central nervous system, which in turn blocked pain.

Dr. Kirkaldy-Willis' conclusion from the study was: "The physician who makes use of this [manipulation] resource will provide relief for many back pain patients."

In 1990, Dr. TW Meade published the results of a randomized comparison of chiropractic and hospital outpatient treatment in the treatment of low back pain. This trial involved 741 patients and was published in the prestigious British Medical Journal (10). It was titled:

Low back pain of mechanical origin: Randomized comparison of chiropractic and hospital outpatient treatment

The patients in this studied were followed for a period between 1 – 3 years. Nearly all of the chiropractic management involved traditional joint manipulation. Key points presented in this article include: "Chiropractic treatment was more effective than hospital outpatient management, mainly for patients with chronic or severe back pain."

"There is, therefore, economic support for use of chiropractic in low back pain, though the obvious clinical improvement in pain and disability attributable to chiropractic treatment is in itself an adequate reason for considering the use of chiropractic."

"Chiropractic was particularly effective in those with fairly intractable pain-that is, those with a history of severe pain."

"Patients treated by chiropractors were not only no worse off than those treated in hospital but almost certainly fared considerably better and that they maintained their improvement for at least two years."

"The results leave little doubt that chiropractic is more effective than conventional hospital outpatient treatment."

Most importantly, the above studies indicate that the primary tissue origin of chronic back pain is the intervertebral disc.

This study by Meade notes that the benefit of chiropractic is seen primarily in patients that are suffering from severe chronic pain.

This would suggest that chiropractic manipulation is affecting the pain afferents arising from the disc. A plausible theory to support this is found below... at the end of this presentation.

Also, the Meade study authors definitively note that if all back pain patients without manipulation contraindications were referred for chiropractic instead of hospital treatment, there would be significant annual treatment cost reductions, a significant reduction in sickness days during the following two years, and a significant savings in social security payments.

In 2003, the highly regarded orthopedic journal SPINE published a randomized clinical trial involving the nonsteroidal anti-inflammatory cox-2 inhibiting drugs Vioxx or Celebrex v. needle acupuncture v. chiropractic manipulation in the treatment of chronic neck and back pain (11). The title of the article is: Chronic Spinal Pain: A Randomized Clinical Trial Comparing Medication, Acupuncture, and Spinal Manipulation

In this study chiropractic was over 5 times more effective than the medications and better than twice as effective as needle acupuncture in the treatment of chronic spine pain.

Chiropractic was able to accomplish these clinical outcomes without any reported adverse effects.

One year after the completion of this 9-week clinical trial, 90% of the original trial participants were re-evaluated to assess their clinical status.

The authors discovered that only those who received chiropractic during the initial randomization benefited from a long-term stable clinical outcome. The results of this second assessment were published in 2005 (12).

An important question to consider...How does joint manipulation reduce chronic back pain arising from the intervertebral disc?

I find that the most plausible explanation is offered by Canadian orthopedic surgeon WH Kirkaldy-Willis in the first edition (1983) of his book titled Managing Low Back Pain .

Dr. Kirkaldy-Willis describes the biomechanics of how the two facet joints form a three-joint complex with the intervertebral disc.

He notes that "motion at one site must reflect motion at the other two." It is probable that spinal manipulation primarily mechanically affects the facet articulations.

According to Dr. Kirkaldy-Willis, such facet motion would necessarily cause motion in the intervertebral disc. Consistent with the published data noted above, this would improve fluid mechanics of the disc, disperse the accumulation of inflammatory exudates, and initiate a neurological sequence of events that would "close the pain gait."

In the final conclusion, the outcomes of the clinical trials noted speak for themselves.

Low Back Pain and Sleep

Low **back pain** (LBP) can arise from a lot of causes, most commonly from bending, lifting, pulling, pushing, and twisting. However, there are other possible causes, including sleep. This not only includes sleeping in a crooked or faulty position, such as falling asleep on a couch, in a chair or while riding in a car, but also from the lack of sleep. So the question is, how much sleep is needed to feel restored and how much sleep is needed to avoid low back pain?

It's been shown that the lack of sleep, or chronic sleep loss, can lead to serious diseases including (but not limited to): heart disease, heart attack, heart failure, irregular heartbeat, high blood pressure, stroke and diabetes. Sleepiness can also result in a disaster; as was the case in the 1979 nuclear accident at Three Mile Island, the oil spill from the Exxon Valdez, as well as the 1986 nuclear disaster at Chernobyl. With sleep deprivation, our reaction time is slowed down, and hence, driving safety is a major issue. The National Highway Traffic Safety Administration estimates that fatigue causes more than 100,000 crashes per year with 1500 annual crash-related deaths in the US alone. This problem is greatest in people under 25 years old. Job related injuries are also reportedly more frequently, especially repeat injuries in workers complaining of daytime sleepiness which resulted in more sick days. It's also well published that sleep plays a crucial role in thinking and learning. Lack of sleep impairs concentration, attention, alertness, reasoning, and general cognitive function. In essence, it makes it more difficult to learn efficiently. Also, getting into a deep sleep cycle plays a critical role in "consolidating memories" in the brain, so if you don't get to a deep sleep stage (about 4 hours of uninterrupted sleep), it's more difficult to remember what you've learned. An interesting study (U. of Pennsylvania) reported that people who slept less than 5 hours/night for 7 nights felt stressed, angry, sad, and mentally exhausted. As shown in another study of 10,000 people, over time, insomnia (the lack of sleep) increases the chances by 5-fold for developing clinical depression. Other clinical studies have published many other negative effects of sleep deprivation, of which some include aging of the skin, forgetfulness, weight gain, and more.

Regarding low back pain, what comes first? Does LBP cause sleep interference or does sleep deprivation cause the LBP (or both)? It's been shown that sleep loss can lower your pain threshold and pain tolerance, making any existing pain feel worse, so it works both ways. Specific to LBP, in a 28-year, 902 metal industry worker study, sleep disturbances (insomnia and/or nightmares) predicted a 2.1-fold increase in back pain hospitalizations with one and a 2.4-fold increase with both sleep disturbance causes (insomnia and nightmares). Other studies have shown patients with chronic LBP had less restful sleep and more "alpha EEG" sleep compared to controls. Similar sleep pattern differences using EEG (electroencephalogram – measures brain waves) have been shown when comparing chronic LBP patients with vs. without depression compared to controls (non-LBP, non-depressed subjects).

So the BOTTOM LINE, talk to us about how chiropractic helps reduce LBP, stress and facilitates sleep. There are also nutritional benefits from Melatonin, valarian root, and others that we can discuss. Now, go to bed and get a good night's sleep!

Low Back Pain and Sleep – Part 2

Last month, we discussed the relationship between sleep deprivation and low **back pain** (LBP) and found that LBP can cause sleep loss AND sleep loss can cause LBP. It's a 2-way street! This month, we will look at ways to improve your sleep quality, which in return, will reduce your LBP. There are many ways we can improve our sleep quality. Here are some of them:

1. Turn off the lights: Complete darkness (or as close to it as possible) is best. Even the tiniest bit of light in the room can disrupt your internal clock and your pineal gland's production of melatonin and serotonin. Cover your windows with blackout shades or drapes.
2. Stay cool! The bedroom's temperature should be =70 degrees F (21 degrees C). At about four hours after you fall asleep, your body's internal temperature drops to its lowest level. Scientists report a cooler bedroom mimics your body's natural temperature drop.
3. Move the alarm clock. Keeping it out of reach (at least 3 feet) forces you to get out of bed and get moving in the AM. Also, you won't be inclined to stare at it during the night!
4. Avoid loud alarm clocks. It is very stressful on your body to be suddenly jolted awake. If you are

114

regularly getting enough sleep, an alarm may even be unnecessary.

5. Reserve your bed for sleeping. Avoid watching TV or doing work in bed, you may find it harder to relax and drift off to sleep.

6. Get to bed before 11pm. Your adrenal system does a majority of its recharging between the hours of 11 p.m. and 1 a.m. and adrenal "burn-out" results in fatigue and other problems.

7. Be consistent about your bed time. Try to go to bed and wake up at the same times each day, including weekends. This will help your body to get into a sleep rhythm and make it easier to fall asleep and get up in the morning.

8. Establish a bedtime routine. Consider meditation, deep breathing, using aromatherapy, or essential oils, or massage from your partner. Relax and reduce your tension from the day.

9. Eat a high-protein snack several hours before bed to provide the L-tryptophan needed for your melatonin and serotonin production.

There are other "tricks" that ensure a good night's rest that we will continue with next month as this is a VERY important subject and can literally add years to your life and life to your years.

Low Back Pain and Sleep – Part 3

For the last 2 months, we've discussed the importance of sleep and its effect on low **back pain** (LBP). Last month, we offered 9 ways to improve sleep quality, and this month we will conclude this topic with 11 more. Sleep deprivation has been called, "…an epidemic" by the Centers for Disease Control and Prevention. To achieve and maintain good health, we must ensure restorative sleep! Here are additional ways to do that (continued from last month):

1. Avoid snacks at bedtime …especially grains and sugars as these will raise your blood sugar and delay sleep. Later, when blood sugar drops too low (hypoglycemia), you not only wake up but falling back to sleep becomes problematic. Dairy foods can also interrupt sleep.
2. Take a hot bath, shower or sauna before bed. This will raise your body temperature and cooling off facilitates sleep. The temperature drop from getting out of the bath signals to your body that "it's time for bed."
3. Keep your feet warm! Consider wearing socks to bed as our feet often feel cold before the rest of the body because they have the poorest circulation. Cold feet make falling asleep difficult!
4. Rest your mind! Stop "brain work" at least 1 hour before bed to give your mind a rest so you can calm down. Don't think about tomorrow's schedule or deadlines.
5. Avoid TV right before bed. TV can be too stimulating to the brain, preventing you from falling asleep quickly as it disrupts your pineal gland function.
6. Consider a "sound machine." Listen to the sound of white noise or nature sounds, such as the ocean or forest, to drown out upsetting background noise and soothe you to sleep.
7. Relaxation reading. Don't read anything stimulating, such as a mystery or suspense novels, as it makes sleeping a challenge.
8. Avoid PM caffeine. Studies show that caffeine can stay active in your system long after consumption.
9. Avoid alcohol. Though drowsiness can occur, many will often wake up several hours later, unable to fall

back asleep. This can prohibit deep sleep, the most restoring sleep (~4th hour).
10. Exercise regularly! Exercising for at least 30 minutes per day can improve your sleep.
11. Increase your melatonin. If you can't increase levels naturally with exposure to bright sunlight in the daytime and absolute complete darkness at night, consider supplementation.

Low Back Pain: What Are Your Treatment Goals?

Low **back pain** (LBP) has been a challenge to treat for centuries and evidence exists that back pain has been a concern since the origins of man. Chiropractic offers one of the most patient satisfying and fastest treatment approaches available. But, when you go to a chiropractor, there seems to be a lot of different approaches utilized from doctor to doctor. Is there any evidence that suggests one approach is favored over another? How are the patient's goals addressed?

Let's look at what chiropractors actually do. Sure, we manipulate the spine and other joints in the upper and lower limbs using a variety of techniques, which seems to be the "brand" of chiropractic. This is good as joint manipulation has consistently been reported to be safe, effective, and with few side effects. Since this is the "staple" of chiropractic, it's safe to say that regardless of our preferred or chosen technique, obtaining a good result is highly likely.

But, chiropractic includes SO MUCH MORE than just joint manipulation! For example, we focus on the whole person, not just their isolated issue or complaint. Using low back pain as our example, a "typical" evaluation includes a detailed history of the patient's general health, past history, illness history, family history, personal habits including sleep quality, exercise habits, dietary issues, quality of life measurements and a review of systems. By gathering this information, we can identify areas that may be directly related to low back pain care, indirectly related, or possibly not related at all, but interferes with the person's quality of life which, in turn, increases LBP. It's really difficult to separate our low back from the rest of our body.

For example, if a person has plantar fasciitis, a heel spur, an ingrown toe nail, diabetic neuropathy in their feet, pes planus or flat feet, an unstable ankle from multiple sprains, knee or hip problems, the gait pattern or, the way a person walks will be affected and the "domino effect" can trickle up to change the low back/pelvic function — resulting in low back pain! Proper management must address all of the issues that are affecting the patient's gait if long-term success in low back pain management is expected, rather than just putting a "band aid" on the problem.

Let's talk about what treatment goals we like to address when we treat our low back pain patient population. The most obvious first goal is pain cessation or getting rid of pain! Since this is what usually drives the patient into our office, patient satisfaction with the care received will not be significant unless the pain is managed. This is achieved through advice, reassurance and training. We often recommend ice (vs. heat) aimed at reducing inflammation, activity modification (teaching proper bending, lifting, pulling, and pushing techniques) and gentle stretching exercises when LBP is present in this acute stage.

Once the pain becomes more manageable and activities become less limited, the second goal is structural restoration. This usually includes managing the flat foot possibly with foot orthotics, a short leg with a heel lift, sole lift or combination, an unstable ankle, knee or hip with exercise often emphasizing balance challenge exercises, and sometimes an orthotic that can be as simple as an elastic wrap to a more elaborate brace. This goal also includes "functional restoration" or transitioning the patient back into real life activities they may be afraid to try such as work, golf, gardening, walking or running, etc.

The third goal is prevention oriented. This may include nutrition (including vitamin/mineral recommendations), weight management (though this is also part of the 2nd goal), exercises (aerobic, stabilization, balance, stretch), and stress management (yoga, lifestyle coaching, etc.). We treat ALL of you, not just your parts!

Low Back and Leg Pain – Is it Sciatica?

Low **back pain** (LBP) can be localized and contained to only the low back area or, it can radiate pain down the leg. This distinction is important as the former, LBP only, is often less complicated and carries a more favorable prognosis for complete recovery. In fact, a large part of our history and examination is focused at this differentiation. This month's Health Update is going to look at the different types of leg pain that can occur with different LBP conditions.

We've all heard of the word "sciatica" and it (usually) is loosely used to describe everything from LBP arising from the joints in the back, the sacroiliac joint, from the muscles of the low back as well as a pinched nerve from a ruptured disk. Strictly speaking, the term "sciatica" should ONLY be used when the sciatic nerve is pinched. The sciatic nerve is made up of five smaller nerves (L4, 5, S1, 2, 3) that arise from the spine and join together to form one large nerve (about the size of our pinky) called the sciatic nerve – like five small rivers merging into one BIG river. Sciatica occurs when any one of the small nerves (L4-S3) or, when the sciatic nerve itself, gets compressed or irritated. This can be, and often is caused from a lumbar disk herniation (the "ruptured disk"), a mis-positioned vertebra (such as a forward slip of the vertebra called "spondylolisthesis"), pressure from an arthritic spur off the spine where the nerve exits ("spinal stenosis"), or, from a tumor near or around the nerve. A term called "pseudo sciatica" (a non-disk cause) includes a pinch from the piriformis muscle where the nerve passes through the pelvis (in the "cheek" or, the buttocks), which has been commonly referred to as "wallet sciatica" as sitting on the wallet in the back pocket is often the cause. When this occurs, the term "peripheral neuropathy" is the most accurate term to use. Other "pseudo sciatic" causes include referred pain from the facet joints which is described by the patient as a "deep ache" inside the leg, or from a metabolic condition where the nerve is affected such as diabetes and other conditions. Here again, the term, "neuropathy" is the better label when diabetes, hypothyroid, lead poisoning, alcohol toxicity and/or others is the culprit. Direct trauma like a bruise to the buttocks from falling or hitting the nerve during an injection into the buttocks can also trigger "sciatica."

The symptoms of sciatica include low back pain, buttocks pain, back of the thigh, calf and/or foot pain and/or numbness-tingling. If the nerve is compressed hard enough, muscle weakness can occur making it hard to stand up on the tip toes creating a limp when walking. In the clinic, we will raise the straight leg and if pinched, sharp pain can occur with as little as 20-30° due to the nerve being stretched as the leg is raised. If pain occurs anywhere between 30 and 70° of elevation of either the same side leg and/or the opposite leg, this constitutes a positive test for sciatica (better termed, "nerve root tension"). When a disk is herniated into the nerve, bending the spine backwards can move the disk away and off the nerve resulting in relief, which is very diagnostic of a herniated disk. Having a patient walk on their toes and then heels and watching for foot drop as well as testing the reflexes, the sensation with a sharp object, and testing the reflexes at the knee and Achilles tendon can give us clues if there is nerve damage. The GOOD NEWS is that chiropractic methods can resolve this problem FREQUENTLY, thus avoiding unnecessary surgery! So, check with us FIRST, before electing for surgery!!!

Is It My Low Back Or My Hip?

When patients present with low **back pain**, it is not uncommon for pain to arise from areas other than the low back, such as the hip. There are many tissues in the low back and hip region that are susceptible to injury with have overlapping pain pathways that often make it challenging to isolate the truly injured area. Hip pain can present in many different ways.

When considering the anatomy of the low back (lumbar spine) and hip, and the nerves that innervate the hip come from the low back, it's no wonder that differentiating between the two conditions is often difficult. Complaints may include the inside, outside, front or back of the thigh, the knee, the buttocks, the sacroiliac joint, or the low back and yet, the hip may truly be the pain generator with any of these presentations. To make diagnosis even more complex, the hip pain patient may present one day with what appears to be sciatic nerve pain (that is, pain shooting down the back of the leg to the knee if mild or, to the foot if more severe) but the next time, with only groin pain. When pain radiates down a leg, the almost automatic impression by both the patient and the health care provider is, "…it's a pinched nerve." But again, it could be the hip and NOT a pinched nerve that is creating the leg pain pattern. Throwing yet another wrench in the works is the fact that a patient can have more than one condition at the same time. So, they truly MAY simultaneously have BOTH a low back problem AND a hip problem. In fact, it's actually unusual to x-ray the low back of a hip pain patient without seeing some low back condition(s) like degenerative disk disease, osteoarthritis (spurs off the vertebrae), or combination of these. So, how do we differentiate between hip vs. low back pain when it is common for both low back and hip pain to often coincide?

During our history, we often ask the question, "…what activities make your pain worse?" If the patient replies that weight bearing activities like standing, walking, getting up from sitting, etc., provoke the pain (and they point to the front or side of the hip), a hip related diagnosis is favored but, it STILL may be arising from the low back or both! If they say, "…crossing my right leg over the other hurts in my groin," that's getting more hip pain specific as hip rotation is frequently lost before the forward flexion motion. When we ask the hip pain patient to point to the area of greatest discomfort, they usually point to the front of the hip or groin, and less often to the inner and/or anterior thigh or knee. Non-weight bearing positions like sitting or lying are almost always immediately pain relieving. When there is arthritis in the hip, motion loss is often reported and may include a shorter walking stride and pain usually gets worse the longer these patients are on their feet. Initiating motion often hurts, sometimes even in bed when rolling over. During the chiropractic examination, with the patient lying on the back with the knee and hip both bent 90°, moving the bent knee outwards or inwards will almost always reproduce hip/groin area pain. Pulling on or, applying traction to the affected leg usually, "…feels good." Knee & ankle reflexes and sensation are normal but muscle strength may be weak due to pain. Bending the low back into different positions does not reproduce pain if the pain is only coming from the hip. Though challenging sometimes, we are well trained to be able to differentiate between hip and low back pain and will treat both areas when it is appropriate.

Demand Soars For Back Pain Treatment After Doctor Makes Refreshing Pledge

What Every Back pain and Herniated Disc Sufferer Should Know About Treatment Options and Choosing A Doctor That Is Right For You

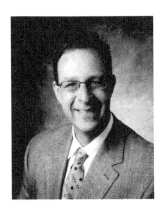

Lacey / Olympia – If you suffer with back pain, you probably already been to many doctors and tried several treatments…without great results.

Or maybe your back pain is new and you don't know who to listen to. There are so many different treatments and "opinions," it can be extremely frustrating. Even worse, if you have been told you have a herniated disc – the pain can be excruciating and the thought of facing back surgery can be terrifying.

What Are The Best Options? Thankfully, research has been done that helps solve some this puzzle – and give

124

you some of the answers you are looking for. And now research has shown one treatment to be both safe and effective for many cases of low back pain in patients with lumbar herniated discs.

But before we talk about this treatment – please understand this... What you are about to discover is a REAL treatments performed by qualified doctors. This is NOT some "wonder cure" you see on Facebook or late night TV.

Here is the important truth: There is no 100% guaranteed cure for back pain with or without a herniated disc. No ethical doctor would ever guarantee results or lead you to believe they have a 100% cure for back pain. But there is a treatment that has already helped countless back pain sufferers...possibly just like you.

In fact, here is what researchers said about this treatment in a 2014 study published in Journal of Manipulative and Physiological Therapeutics: *"The proportion of patients reporting clinically relevant improvement in this current study is surprisingly good, with nearly 70% of patients improved as early as 2 weeks after the start of treatment. By 3 months, this figure was up to 90.5% and then stabilized at 6 months and 1 year."*

We will get into more proof in just a bit…but here is something you should know first…because the treatment is only as good as the doctor you choose…

There is a doctor using this treatment that has taken a very refreshing pledge that has led to back pain sufferers flocking to his office.

This doctor's name is Dr. David Warwick and he is a Chiropractor in Lacey/Olympia WA.

Here Is Something Extremely Important – You may have already been to a Chiropractor or just heard some things you did not like. So…Why is this Chiropractor different and why are so many back pain sufferers willing to give him a try – even when they have been to many other doctors already?

The answer is simple…Dr. Warwick took this pledge…"To the best of my ability, I agree to provide my patient's convenient, affordable, and mainstream Chiropractic care. I will not use unnecessary long-term treatment plans and/or therapies."

In other words, Dr. Warwick uses treatments that are widely accepted and has a goal to treat patients the least amount of times possible. For this reason, Dr. Warwick NEVER tries to sell you a multiple visit, long term treatment plan that can cost thousands of dollars.

Instead, Dr. Warwick does something his patients absolutely love – he accepts patients on a visit-by-visit basis. In other words, he treats you once and you decide if it is something you like and want to continue. There is no commitment and seeing patients as little as possible has made care extremely affordable – even if you do not have insurance coverage.

This no pressure, patient first approach is so refreshing, it has patients rant and raving...and the referrals have come in droves.

There is also one other thing about Dr. Warwick patients love...Because he is mainstream, he works hand-in-hand with his colleagues in the medical community. Dr. Warwick gives and receives referrals from the medical doctors all the time because his goal is to give the patient (you) exactly what you want and is best for you.

What Is The Treatment And Is There Any Proof? The treatment is spinal manipulative therapy – and if you have back pain – you are going to love this...

We have already mentioned one quote from the 2014 study...here is another..."This study shows that patients with proven lumbar intervertebral disc herniation and compressive neuropathology that receive traditional chiropractic side-posture manipulation are both safe and effective. The ultimate clinical effectiveness of about 90%

is impressive when compared to any form of therapy, and with no reported serious side effects.

This study would suggest that all patients suffering from lumbar intervertebral disc herniation with compressive neuropathology should be treated with chiropractic spinal adjusting."

Is It Safe? According to the study…"Spinal Manipulative Therapy is a very safe and cost effective option for treating symptomatic lumbar disc herniation."

Dr. Warwick is 100% honest and he would like you to know this: Research helps doctors help patients – but no one should expect the results from this study or any other study. All patients are different and all cases are individual. That's why treatment outcomes can never be predicted for any one person. This is why Dr. Warwick offers treatment with no long term commitment – so you can give it a try and see if it works for you.

Who Should Try This Treatment With Dr. Warwick? You may be a good candidate if you have: (1) Acute low back pain with or without leg pain, (2) low back pain with a herniated or bulging disc – with or without leg pain, (3) chronic low back pain.

It is important to note that, according to the study, "Even the chronic patients in this study, with the mean duration of their symptoms being over 450 days, reported significant improvement, although this takes slightly longer."

Dr. Warwick's Invitation To You – Dr. Warwick offers a limited number of complimentary consultations every month. The purpose is to see if you are a good candidate for this treatment...and so you can get your questions answered. If you would like a complimentary consultation with Dr. Warwick, just **CALL 360-951-4504 or VISIT** DrDavidWarwick.com for convenient on-line scheduling. The best thing about the consultation is you will feel relieved finally getting some straight answers about your back pain and the best course of action.

Low Back Pain & Spinal Manipulation: How Does It Work?

For many years, Chiropractic has been at the forefront of treating low **back pain** (LBP) with both greater patient satisfaction and less lost time at work when compared to other non-surgical treatment approaches. There have been many explanations as to why chiropractic manipulation therapy (CMT) works but many of these studies include other treatment modalities or methods and the benefits are ,therefore, not clearly derived only from CMT. A recent study has tried to clear this up and the results are very interesting!

This study included two chiropractors and two a physical therapists (PT) from Canada and the US. What is unique about this study is that they measured clinical or symptomatic improvement by tracking improvement in activity tolerance using a standard questionnaire commonly used by chiropractors and PTs all over the world, as well as changes in the spinal stiffness using a valid/reliable instrument before and after CMT was utilized. The importance of these findings is that only CMT was utilized and hence, other forms of treatment commonly utilized by chiropractors did not cloud the findings. There were 48 patients included in the study and the initial 2 treatments were administered 3-4 days apart, followed by an assessment 3-4 days after the 2nd treatment. Assessments were also performed before and after each treatment. The assessments included use of the questionnaire and a stiffness measurement using the special instrument. Also, "recruitment of the lumbar multifidus muscle" (a muscle in the low back that helps stabilize the trunk or core) was measured by ultrasound. After each treatment, significant improvement was found in the overall pain level and in reduced spinal stiffness (which remained improved 3-4 days after the last/second treatment).

The study conclusions revealed less pain, more activity tolerance and less spinal stiffness after the administration of the 2 treatments. The greatest clinical improvement was found in those who had the most dramatic reduction in stiffness after each treatment. They found that the level of muscle recruitment was directly related to the degree of spinal stiffness. They also found that patients who received thrust manipulation (CMT) had immediate improvements with reduced pain, stiffness and improved muscle recruitment measurements. However, this same effect was NOT obtained when non-thrust mobilization techniques were used. This means many non-thrust manual techniques such as mobilization, massage, and other soft tissue release methods do not create the immediate benefits that were produced by thrust manipulation.

With this new information, we are now able to explain with confidence to patients the reasons why they typically feel better after the spinal adjustment. The patient can then appreciate receiving an answer that makes clear sense and has been "proven." It's important to realize that the "bonus" of receiving chiropractic care for low back pain includes not only just pain reduction, but more importantly, improvement in tolerating activities such as vacuuming, washing dishes, golfing, walking and of course, working

Low Back Pain: Spondylolisthesis

Low **back pain** can arise from many conditions, one of which is a mouthful: spondylolisthesis. The term was coined in 1854 from the Greek words, "spondylo" for vertebrae and "olisthesis" for slip. These "slips" most commonly occur in the low back, 90% at L5 and 9% at L4. According to www.spinehealth.com and others, the most common type of spondylolisthesis is called "isthmic spondylolisthesis," which is a condition that includes a defect in the back part of the vertebra in an area called the pars interarticularis, which is the part of the vertebra that connects the front half (vertebral body) to the back half (the posterior arch). This can occur on one, or both sides, with or without a slip or shift forwards, which is then called spondylolysis. In "isthmic spondylolisthesis," the incidence rate is about 5-7% of the general population favoring men over women 3:1. Debate continues as to whether this occurs as a result genetic predisposition verses environmental or acquired at some point early in life as noted by the increased incidence in populations such as Eskimos (30-50%), where they traditionally carry their young in papooses, vertically loading their lower spine at a very young age. However, isthmic spondylolisthesis can occur at any time in life if a significant backward bending force occurs resulting in a fracture but reportedly, occurs most frequently between ages 6 and 16 years old.

Often, traumatic isthmic spondylolisthesis occurs during the adolescent years and in fact, is the most common cause of low back pain at this stage of life. Sports most commonly resulting in spondylolisthesis include gymnastics, football (lineman), weightlifting (from squats or dead lifts) and diving (from overarching the back). Excessive backward bending is the force that overloads the back of the vertebra resulting in the fracture sometimes referred to as a stress fracture, which is a fracture that occurs as a result of repetitive overloading over time, usually weeks to months.

If the spondylolisthesis lesions do not heal either by cartilage or by bone replacement, the front half of the vertebra can slip or slide forwards and become unstable. Fortunately, most of these heal and become stable and don't progress. The diagnosis is a simple x-ray, but to determine the degree of stability, "stress x-rays" or x-rays taken at endpoints of bending over and backwards are needed. Sometimes, a bone scan is needed to determine if it's a new injury verses an old isthmic spondylolisthesis.

Another very common type is called degenerative spondylolisthesis and occurs in 30% of Caucasian and 60% of African-American woman (3:1 women to men). This usually occurs at L4 and is more prevalent in aging females. It is sometimes referred to as "pseudospondylolisthesis" as it does not include defects in the posterior arch but rather, results from a degeneration of the disk and facet joints. As the disk space narrows, the vertebra slides forwards. The problem here is that the spinal canal, where the spinal cord travels, gets crimped or distorted by the forward sliding vertebra and causes compression of the spinal nerve root(s), resulting pain and/or numbness in one or both legs. The good news about spondylolisthesis is that non-surgical approaches, like spinal manipulation in particular, work well and chiropractic is a logical treatment approach!

Where Is My Pain Coming From?

Low **back pain** can emanate from many anatomical locations (as well as a combination of locations), which always makes it interesting when a patient asks, "…doc, where in my back is my pain coming from?" In context of an office visit, we take an accurate history and perform our physical exam to try to reproduce symptoms to give us clues as to what tissue(s) may be the primary pain generators. In spite of our strong intent to be accurate, did you know, regardless of the doctor type, there is only about a 45% accuracy rate when making a low back pain diagnosis? This is partially because there are many tissues that can be damaged or injured that are innervated by the same nerve fibers and hence, clinically they look very similar to each other. In order to improve this rather sad statistic, in 1995 the Quebec Task Force published research reporting that accuracy could be improved to over 90% if we utilize a classification approach where low back conditions are divided into 1 of 3 broad categories:

1. Red flags – These include dangerous conditions such as cancer, infection, fracture, cauda equine syndrome (which is a severe neurological condition where bowel and bladder function is impaired). These conditions generally require emergency care due to the life threatening and/or surgical potential.
2. Mechanical back pain – These diagnoses include facet syndromes, ligament and joint capsule sprains, muscle strains, degenerative joint disease (also called osteoarthritis), and spondylolisthesis.
3. Nerve Root compression – These conditions include pinching of the nerve roots, most frequently from herniated disks. This category can include spinal stenosis (SS) or, combinations of both, but if severe enough where the spinal cord is compromised (more commonly in the neck), SS might then be placed in the 1st of the 3 categories described above.

The most common category is mechanical back pain of which "facet syndrome" is the most common condition. This is the classic patient who over did it ("The Weekend Warrior") and can hardly get out of bed the next day. These conditions can include tearing or stretching of the capsule surrounding the facet joint due to performing too many bending, lifting, or twisting related activities. The back pain is usually localized to the area of injury but can radiate down into the buttocks or back of the thigh and can be mild to very severe.

Low Back Pain: Why Is It So Common?

This question has plagued all of us, including researchers for a long time! Could it be because we're all inherently lazy and don't exercise enough? Or maybe it's because we have a job that's too demanding on our back? To properly address this question, here are some interesting facts:

1. The prevalence of low **back pain** (LBP) is common, as 70-85% of ALL PEOPLE have back pain that requires treatment of some sort at some time in life.
2. On a yearly basis, the annual prevalence of back pain averages 30% and once you have back pain, the likelihood of recurrence is high.
3. Back pain is the most common cause of activity limitation in people less than 45 years of age.
4. Back pain is the 2nd most frequent reason for physician visits, the 5th ranking reason for hospital admissions, and is the 3rd most common cause for surgical procedures.
5. About 2% of the US workforce receives compensation for back injuries annually.
6. Similar statistics exist for other countries, including the UK and Sweden.

So, what are the common links as to why back pain is so common? One reason has to do with the biomechanics of the biped – that is, the two legged animal. When compared to the 4-legged species, the vertically loaded spine carries more weight in the low back, shows disk and joint deterioration and/or arthritis much sooner, and we overload the back more frequently because, well, we can! We have 2 free arms to lift and carry items that often weigh way too much for our back to be able to safely handle. We also lift and carry using poor technique. Another reason is anatomical as the blood supply to our disks is poor at best, and becomes virtually non-existent after age 30. That makes healing of disk tears or cracks nearly impossible. Risk factors for increased back injury include heavy manual lifting requirements, poor or low control of the work environment, and prior incidence of low back pain. Other risk factors include psychosocial issues such as fear of injury, beliefs that pain means one should not work, beliefs that treatment or time will not help resolve a back episode, the inability to control the condition, high anxiety and/or depression levels, and more. Because there are so many reasons back problems exist, since the early 1990's, it has been strongly encouraged that we as health care providers utilize a "biopsychosocial model" of managing those suffering with low back pain, which requires not only treatment but proper patient education putting to rest unnecessary fears about back pain.

Low Back Pain and Spinal Fusions

You may think it's odd to discuss low **back pain** (LBP) from the perspective of spinal fusion because as chiropractors, we do not perform surgery and so, why discuss it? It is important that we discuss research such as this so we can make the informed treatment decisions with our patients after we've considered all the facts in each specific case. Now, there are certainly times when a surgical procedure for back and leg pain is necessary and appropriate for some patients, but the problem is, there are also some patients who have been told they need spinal surgery when, in fact, they may be better off NOT proceeding with surgery. So, the question is, what happens to those patients who elect not, vs. those who do choose to proceed with surgery?

That question was addressed in a study where a total of 1450 patients injured at work were followed over a 2-year time frame. There were a total of 725 patients who proceeded with the fusion surgery and the other 750 elected NOT to have the surgery. A fusion surgery can be described as when two or more vertebra are fused together, usually because there are neurological problems such as shooting leg pain, weakness and/or numbness in one or both legs. The conditions treated in this study included herniated disks, degeneration of the disk, and radiating leg pain. There were primarily 3 factors that were compared between the two groups, namely, 1) ability to return to work; 2) disability (the inability to work), and 3) opiate (narcotic) drug use. Other factors compared included the need for re-operations, complications, and death.

The results showed, in general, those who proceeded with surgery had significantly more problems compared to those who did not have surgery. For example, only 26% returned to work, compared to 67% returned to work. The total number of days off work were 1140 vs. 316 days, respectively. There were 17 vs. 11 deaths, respectively and, 27% of the surgical group required re-operations with a 36% complication rate. Also, there was a 41% increase in the use of narcotic medication with 76% continuing the use after surgery.

Again, there are times when surgery is absolutely the right choice. Those times include when there is a loss of bladder or bowel control, progressively worsening neurological symptoms in spite of non-surgical care, and of course, unstable fractures, cancer/tumor and infections, but that's about it! In other words, if you don't have one of the before mentioned conditions which do require surgery, don't be too quick to jump at the chance of "getting it fixed" with surgery. As the study suggests, the post-surgical results favor those who elected NOT to have surgery. Also, when in doubt, don't trust the opinion of only one surgeon – always get a 2nd or even 3rd opinion. It is also very important to consider your current level of function or, your ability to do your desired tasks and, unless there is a significant loss in that ability, consider additional time with non-surgical treatment. The non-surgical treatment you can expect to receive from chiropractic includes (but may not be limited to) spinal manipulation, exercise training, physical therapy modalities (ice, heat, electrical stimulation, ultrasound, traction, etc.), dietary counseling, and job modification information.

Low Back Pain and Balance Exercises

You may recall last month, we talked about the relationship between low **back pain** and balance, particularly our unfortunate increased tendency to fall as we "mature." This month, we're going to look at ways to improve our balance by learning specific exercises that utilize the parts of our nervous system that regulate balance or, proprioception. Particularly, our cerebellum (back of the brain that regulates coordination), the vestibular system (the inner ear where the semi-circular canals are located), the ascending tracts in our spinal cord (the "highways" that bring information to the brain from our feet and the rest of our body), and the small "mechano-receptors" located in our joints that pick up our movements as we walk and run and sends that information through our nerves, up the spinal cord tracts to the brain. Here are some very practical exercises to do, "...for the rest of our lives." Start with the easy ones!

1. Easy (Level 1) : Standing eyes open/closed – Start with the feet shoulder width apart, look straight ahead to get your balance and then close the eyes and try not to sway counting to 30 by, "...one thousand one, one thousand two, one thousand three, etc." Repeat this with your feet closer together until they touch each other. You can make this harder by standing on a pillow or cushion — but don't start that way!

- Medium (Level 2) : Lunges – from a similar starting position as #1, step forwards with one leg and squat slightly before returning back to the start position. Repeat this 5x with each foot/leg. As you progress, you can take a longer stride and/or squat down further with each repetition. You can even hold onto light dumbbells and/or close your eyes to make it more challenging.
- Hard (Level 3) : Rocker or wobble board exercises – use a platform that rocks back & forth or, wobbles in multiple directions. Rock back and forth, eyes open and then closed, once you get comfortable on the board. You can rotate your body on the board, standing straight ahead (12 o'clock) followed by 45 degree angles as you work your way around in a circle at 45 degree increments (12, 1:30, 3, 4:30, 6, 7:30, 9, 10:30 and back to noon). Repeat these eyes open and closed. The Wii Balance board is a fun way to exercise – check that out as well. You can "improvise" and mix up different exercises and create your own routine. Just remember, stay safe, work slowly until you build up your confidence and keep challenging yourself.

Would Traction Help My Back Pain?

Traction is a common form of treatment for patients with low **back pain**. By definition, traction is the "act of pulling a body part." That basically means traction can be applied to an arm, leg, finger, toe… virtually any body part that one can get a hold of. Here, the focus of traction is being applied to the lower part of the spine and the primary objective is for pain relief and restoring function. Traction "works" by applying a force that separates and increases the space between joints. It also stretches the surrounding soft tissues, including ligaments, joint capsules, muscles, and tendons. Spinal traction can be applied manually (with the hands) or by a device with either the use of complicated computerized equipment or by a gravity-assisted means such as using the body's weight and gravity as the traction force.

Common conditions of the spine for which traction is often utilized include low back sprains and strains, disk herniations ("slipped disks"), and spinal stenosis. Spinal stenosis occurs when there is a narrowing of the hole or canal through which a nerve root exits the spine or where the spinal cord travels, often caused by arthritic spurs. Hence, it is most common after the age of 60 years old. Traction has been shown to improve circulation, reduce inflammation, and by movement of the joints, it may also reduce the nerve's excitability, resulting in pain reduction.

The "dose" of traction, from a clinical experience standpoint, is determined by patient comfort. When determining the dose of traction for the first time, patients are advised to pay careful attention to the way they feel during the time traction is applied. Often, it feels good at first but may become uncomfortable as time passes. If there is sharp pain, radiating pain (such as down a leg), or if it is just not comfortable, traction should be discontinued and the recovery time should be reported.

A "typical" dose is 10-15 minutes of time, and the traction force can be continuous or intermittent, kind of like turning on a water faucet and leaving it running vs. turning it on and off. With intermittent traction, your doctor can vary the time that the force is applied such as 30 seconds on and 10 seconds off. Generally, the total treatment time can be longer with intermittent traction (such as 15 minutes) compared to continuous traction, where 10 minutes may be utilized. The traction weight or force can be gradually increased, depending on tolerance and individual patient response to the prior weight.

The Cochrane Report found traction is most effective for cases of sciatica or nerve root pressure creating leg pain. Also, it's best when used in conjunction with other treatment approaches. In a chiropractic setting, manual traction (where the doctor uses their hands to apply the force) is often utilized along with side to side or figure-8 movements to achieve better results. Spinal manipulation, muscles massage, myofascial release techniques, exercise training for both stretch and strengthening purposes, and patient education (such as teaching proper bend/lift/pull/push techniques) are often utilized to achieve the most satisfying results when managing patients with low back pain.

Have You Tried This for Your Back Pain?

It's not uncommon for low back pain patients to reduce their activities in an effort to avoid their pain. Unfortunately, it's likely their core muscles—the muscles that help support their midsection—will become deconditioned over time due to inactivity, which may only increase the risk of further injury. Therefore, to effectively improve one's low back pain status, he or she must first strengthen and keep their core muscles strong! Think in terms of one to three sets of ten reps for ease of application and ALWAYS release the exercise SLOWLY—don't just drop back from the end-range of the exercise.

The ABDOMINAL muscles include four groups: the rectus abdominis (they attach our rib cage to our pelvic area, and the fibers run straight up and down), overlapping on the sides are the internal obliques (fibers run down and inward), the external obliques (fibers run down and out), and lastly, the transverse abdominis (the fibers run horizontal and attach to the fascia in the low back).

If we think of three levels of exercise difficulty, an easy (or Level 1) sit-up can include a "crunch" or simply lifting the head and shoulders off the floor. A more difficult (Level 2) ab exercise would be to bend the knees and hips at 90 degree angles while performing a sit-up, while a more difficult (level 3) ab exercise could be a double straight leg raise during the sit-up. The rectus is stimulated by coming straight up and down while the overlapping obliques require a trunk twist. You can employ an "abdominal brace", or holding the stomach muscles firmly as if someone is going to punch you in the stomach, in any position or activity during the day.

You can strengthen the LOW BACK extensor muscles using a number of effective exercises including (but not limited to) the "bird-dog" (kneeling on "all-fours") straightening the opposite arm and leg separately (Level 1) and then simultaneously and switching back and forth (Level 2). Level 3 could be longer hold times, drawing a square with the hand and foot, or increasing the repetitions.

Another low back strengthener is called the "Superman", which requires laying on the stomach (prone) initially lifting one arm and then the opposite leg separately (Level I); then opposite limbs at the same time (Level 2); and finally raising both arms and legs simultaneously (Level 3). Placing a roll under the pelvis/abdomen can make it more comfortable.

You can strengthen the SIDES OF THE CORE, or lateral trunk stabilizers, using a side-bridge or plank (laying on the side propped up between the elbow and feet, with the hips up and off the floor). Level 1 could be a six-second hold from the knees, Level 2 a six-second hold from the feet, and Level 3 could be a twelve-second hold between the elbow/forearm and feet. A modification could include slow repetitions of lowering the pelvis to the floor and back up. Mix it up!

There are MANY more exercises, but these should keep you going for a while! Remember, stay within "reasonable pain boundaries" that you define, release each exercise SLOWLY, and most importantly, have fun!

The Neck Pain – Headache Connection And What To Do About It Consider…

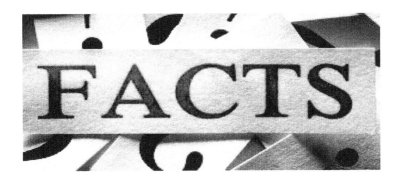

Lacey / Olympia – I'm not a betting person. But here is a safe bet I would take.

If you have neck pain – I'll bet you also suffer with headaches.

It is such a safe bet because doctors that treat both neck pain and headaches know they go hand in hand. In fact, it is probably safe to say that the vast majority of many headache sufferers also have neck pain.

Why is this important for you?

It is important for several reasons. The first is, doctors that treat both headaches and neck pain have also found that the two are not just correlated – they are often connected.

In other words – problems in the neck can and do cause a lot of headaches. In fact, it is so common there is a term for it: "cervicogenic headache."

That's why when patients seek treatment for their headaches, a thorough examination of the neck, upper back, and cranial nerves is routinely performed.

It is common to find upper cervical movement and vertebral alignment problems present in patients complaining of headaches.

These movement and alignment problems are a potential cause of headaches and should be treated for to help both neck pain and headaches.

What's The Best treatment?

Chiropractic manipulation or "adjustments" have been used for over 100 years. Chiropractic manipulations can help correct misalignments and restore proper motion to vertebral segments in your neck.

Chiropractic adjustments applied to the fixated or misaligned vertebra in the upper neck often brings very satisfying relief to the headache sufferer.

Exercises that promote movement in the neck, as well as strengthening exercises are also helpful in both reducing headache pain and in preventing occurrences, especially with stress or tension headaches.

How Long Does It Take To Get Relief?

It is impossible to predict the results of any medical treatment. That's why ethical doctors do not guarantee results.

Every case is individual and it is impossible to predict if this treatment will work for you – and if it does… how long it will take.

But it is not uncommon for some headache sufferers to get relief quickly.

That's why it is important to choose a Chiropractor that offers very flexible treatment plans that does not make you commit to long term treatment plans that can cost thousands of dollars.

It makes more sense to see patients ones visit at a time and see how they are responding to treatment. This way, you can continue if it is working – and you like it – or stop any time you want.

This also makes care very affordable.

If You Want More Help

If you have any question about neck pain and headaches, or would like a free consultation, just CALL Dr. David Warwick at **360-951-4504** or VISIT DrDavidWarwick.com for convenient on-line scheduling. Dr. Warwick is a Chiro-Trust member (For more information, go to www.Chiro-Trust.org) Chiropractor in Lacey who treats neck pain and headaches with treatments that are one visit at a time. He never offers long term, expensive plans. The consultation is 100% free with no further obligation. You will find out if Dr. Warwick can possible help you and get all your questions answered.

What's Better for Neck Pain, Medication or Chiropractic?

Although both medication and chiropractic are utilized by neck pain sufferers, not everyone wants to or can take certain medications due to unwanted side effects. For those who aren't sure what to do, wouldn't it be nice if research was available that could answer the question posted above? Let's take a look!

When people have neck pain, they have options as to where they can go for care. Many seek treatment from their primary care physician (PCP). The PCP's approach to neck pain management usually results in a prescription that may include an anti-inflammatory drug (like ibuprofen or Naproxen), a muscle relaxant (like Flexeril / cyclobenzaprine), and/or a pain pill (like hydrocodone / Vicodin). The choice of which medication a PCP recommends hinges on the patient's presentation, patient preference (driven from advertisements or prior experiences), and/or the PCP's own preference.

Although it's becoming increasingly common to have a PCP refer a neck pain patient for chiropractic care, this still does not happen for all neck pain patients in spite of strong research supporting the significant benefits of spinal manipulation to treat neck pain. One such study compared spinal manipulation, acupuncture, and anti-inflammatory medication with the objective of assessing the long-term benefits (at one year) of these three approaches in patients with chronic (>13 weeks) neck pain. The study randomly divided 115 patients into one of three groups that were all treated for nine weeks. Comparison at the one-year point showed that ONLY those who received spinal manipulation had maintained long-term benefits based on a review of seven main outcome measures. The study concludes that for patients with chronic neck pain, spinal manipulation was the ONLY treatment that maintained a significant long-term (one-year) benefit after nine weeks of treatment!

In a 2012 study published in medical journal The Annals of Internal Medicine, 272 acute or sub-acute neck pain patients received one of three treatment approaches:

medication, exercise with advice from a health care practitioner, or chiropractic care. Participants were treated for twelve weeks, with outcomes assessed at 2, 4, 8, 12, 26, and 52 weeks. The patients in the chiropractic care and exercise groups significantly outperformed the medication group at the 26-week point AND had more than DOUBLE the likelihood of complete neck pain relief. However, at the one-year point, ONLY the chiropractic group continued to demonstrate long-term benefits! The significant benefits achieved from both exercise and chiropractic treatments when compared with medication make sense as both address the cause of neck pain as opposed to only masking the symptoms.

With results of these studies showing acute, subacute, as well as chronic neck pain responding BEST to chiropractic care, it only makes sense to TRY THIS FIRST!

Ever Asked Yourself, "Why Do I Have Neck or Back Pain?"

In a study that looked at stress and how people who seek chiropractic care perceive it, researchers wrote that psychosocial stress, "...pervades modern life and is known to have an impact on health. Pain, especially chronic back pain, is influenced by stress." Here, ten different chiropractic clinics reported results tallied from 138 patients who were given questionnaires about stress and its association with their current condition.

Of interest, more than 30% categorized themselves as being "moderately to severely stressed," and over 50% felt that stress had a moderate or greater effect on their presenting complaint. Further, about 71% of the patients felt that a stress management approach would be useful to help them cope and 44% were interested in taking a "self-development program to enhance their stress management skills."

The study concluded that: 1) patient perceptions are known to be important in management approaches and treatment outcomes; 2) in this study, about 1/3 of patients presenting perceived themselves as being moderately or severely stressed; and 3) interventions that reduce stress or the patient's perception of being stressed may be an important and valid "intervention" in patient management.

So, how do doctors of chiropractic do this? First is pain management, which is often at the core of a current heightened stress level, as it can push the stress level "over the edge." But just managing pain doesn't always work by itself, and doctors of chiropractic will often intervene with nutritional recommendations such as educating the patient about an "anti-inflammatory diet," and the use of vitamin and/or herbal approaches specific to stress management, including specific nutritional approaches to balancing neurotransmitter levels. Other approaches may include the use of various calming techniques that can be employed at times when patients are "stressed" and can be used during the day during these "stressful moments."

There are even "calming apps" to help de-stress and clear the mind available for your smartphone! Just as there are apps to measure your steps, calories, or METS burned during the day, these apps are specific for calming and reducing stress! Here are the names of a few that are FREE for you to investigate and consider (Web, Android, or iOS): MindMeister, Breath2Relax, White Noise Lite, Calm, Diaro, Headspace, Relax, Guided Meditations, and more. Give one of these a try as it is clear we all focus far too little on stress management!

Neck Pain Causes and What To Do

We all know what it feels like to have limited neck motion, as most of us have had neck pain at some point in time. It makes doing simple things like backing up a car, rolling over in bed, reading, and watching TV difficult-to-impossible. The goal of this article is to review some of the many causes of neck pain and what to do about it! Let's take a look at the various types of tissues that can generate pain:

- MUSCLES: There are MANY layers of muscles in the neck. There are the very small, deep "intrinsic" muscles that are important for stability of the spine and fine, intricate movements while the larger outside "extrinsic" muscles are long and strong, allowing us to sustain stresses like playing football, rugby, hockey, or falling on the ice. Long car drives/rides, computer work, studying/reading, or having a conversation with someone not sitting directly in front of you are just a few examples of how these muscles can experience overuse that can generate neck pain!

- LIGAMENTS: These are tough, non-stretching tissues that hold bone to bone and can tear in trauma like whiplash, while playing sports, or in a fall. Because ligaments are important in keeping our joints stable, disrupted ligaments can lead to excessive "play" in a joint and can wear down the cartilage or the smooth, silky covering at the ends of bones, which can lead to premature osteoarthritis (OA) – the "wear and tear" kind that everyone gets eventually.
- WORN JOINTS: There is something called "the natural history of degeneration" that naturally occurs if we live long enough. As previously discussed, ligament tearing leads to instability of the involved joint(s), and excessive motion in the joint leads to OA. In the neck, there are two sets of small joints between six of the seven vertebrae called facet joints and uncinate processes that are vulnerable for OA and are frequent pain generators.
- DISK INJURY: The disks rest between the big vertebral bodies and act as shock absorbers. They are like jelly donuts, and when the disk's tough outer layers tear, the jelly can leak out and this may or may not hurt, depending on the direction, the amount of the leaked out "jelly," and if the "jelly" pinches pain-sensitive tissues. A "herniated disk" is the most common cause for a pinched nerve (see next entry).
- NERVE COMPRESSION: The nerves in the neck travel into the arms, and nerve compression or pinching can result in numbness/tingling/burning pain in the arm and/or hand with or without weakness. Each nerve has a different role, and by mapping the numbness area and testing reflexes and muscle strength, it can help your doctor identify the specific nerve that is injured.
- DISEASES: Though significantly less common, neck pain can arise from certain diseases such as

rheumatoid arthritis, meningitis, and/or cancer. When these are suspect, blood tests and special tests such as bone scan, CT/MRI, and/or biopsy can help to specifically identify the condition.

WHAT TO DO: Make an appointment and your doctor of chiropractic will perform a history, physical examination, and possibly take x-rays to help determine what is generating your pain. Once the diagnosis is understood, he or she will put together a treatment plan for you. This usually includes procedures done in the office as well as those that they will teach you how to do at home and/or work to help you manage your neck pain back and return to normal activities as quickly as possible!

Neck Pain – When Should I Come In?

Neck pain is one of the most common complaints patients have when they come to a chiropractic office for the first time, second only to low back pain. Neck pain affects all of us at some point in life, and for some, it can become a chronic, permanent problem that can interfere with many desired activities and lower their quality of life. There are many different causes, and prompt evaluation and treatment is important is some cases.

Neck pain and stiffness are the two most common symptoms that present for evaluation and treatment. This can be located in the middle of the neck and/or on either side and can extend down to the shoulders and / or chest. It can contribute to or cause tension headaches that can travel up the back of the head and sometimes behind the eyes. Pain often increases with neck movement, such as when turning the head to check traffic while driving and/or it can hurt at rest while held in static positions, such as when reading a book. Neck pain can come on gradually or quickly and often cannot be traced to a specific injury or cause making it a challenge to figure out. While neck pain is often not serious or life-threatening, there are causes that should be evaluated promptly. If you wake up with acute neck pain associated with very limited range of motion, this may be due to torticollis, or wry neck, and prompt treatment helps it resolve more quickly than "waiting it out." Torticollis can be caused by exposure to a draft, changes in weather, trauma, or after a cold or flu. When in doubt, come in for an evaluation and treatment, as anxiety associated with the "fear of the unknown" only adds to the stress associated with neck pain and it's ALWAYS best to be "…safe than sorry!"

Numbness or tingling may accompany neck pain and can be located in the face, arms, hands, and/or fingers. This is one of those times to come in promptly, as these symptoms may indicate the pinching of a nerve root in the neck. There are MANY chiropractic treatment approaches that effectively treat nerve root pinching, and treatment should NOT be delayed. Other common symptoms may include clicking, crunching, or grinding noises, technically called crepitus, which may or may not be benign. If the noise is accompanied by pain, especially if it radiates down to the shoulder blades or arms (either side or both), it's time to promptly come in. Any time symptoms occur acutely or come on fast, it's best to get evaluated as soon as possible.

Dizziness is another common symptom that can result from neck problems and is often associated with movement such as rising from laying or sitting. Certain positions of the neck can also bring on dizziness. This is sometimes caused by the "stones" in the inner ear shifting out of position and is technically called BPPV or "benign paroxysmal positional vertigo." When this occurs, we can usually manage it very well with treatment and specific BPPV exercises. Other times, dizziness may be due to a restriction in blood flow reaching the brain. In which case, a prompt evaluation is VERY appropriate, especially if blackouts occur.

Sleep interruption or difficulty falling asleep are other good reasons to seek prompt evaluation and treatment. Sleep loss can lead to many problems such as excessive fatigue, tiredness, irritability, and just generally feeling poor! Remember, prompt care usually results in prompt resolution!

Chiropractic Management of Neck Pain (Part 1)

Neck pain is a very common condition that drives many patients to seek chiropractic care. Treatment planning typically includes four primary goals: 1) Pain Management; 2) Structural Realignment; 3) Functional Restoration; and 4) Maintenance / Prevention.

1) PAIN MANAGEMENT: Getting rid of pain is the primary focus of ALL patients in the early stages of a neck injury. If we use the acronym "PRICE" (Protect, Rest, Ice, Compress, and Elevate), the first three apply when it comes to neck pain. We "protect" our neck by avoiding or changing the way we go about doing things such as our sleep position (this often prompts a "proper pillow discussion"), adjusting the outside rearview mirrors of our car (if you flair the outside mirrors outwards, it opens up the "blind spots" and may prevent a collision, especially if you cannot rotate your neck very far), and modifying other ADLs (activities of daily living).

The bottom line is: if an activity creates a sharp pain sensation, it is a "warning sign" to modify or stop WHATEVER it is that you're doing. Wearing a cervical collar for a SHORT duration of time can qualify for both "Protect" and "Rest." Try resting your neck on a pillow when reading or watching TV, as it allows the neck muscles to rest. A cervical traction device can help reduce muscle spasm, improves flexibility (range of motion), and reduce pain. Alternating "Ice" and heat can be even more effective, as it "PUMPS" out inflammation or swelling.

Heat is also a good natural muscle relaxant and ice reduces swelling (inflammation), both of which can help reduce pain. There really is no hard and fast rule as to how long you should continue using ice (days, weeks, or months) – if it helps, use it (unless you are hypersensitive and frostbite easily, in which case limit the ice time). However, heat can worsen a condition if it's applied too soon or too long. Anti-inflammatory herbs like ginger, turmeric, boswellia, and others are very effective and actually may be BETTER than ibuprofen, Aleve, or aspirin.

Recent studies indicate that there may be a delay in healing when over-the-counter pain medications are used, and the recommendation is to AVOID these drugs so healing won't be delayed!

2) STRUCTURAL REALIGNMENT: The goal here is to improve (to the best of our ability) faulty bony misalignments that frequently exist in the neck, upper, middle back as well as the low back, as all can contribute to neck pain. This is also a great long-term goal, as it may help PREVENT future episodes of neck pain.

There is a natural process of aging called osteoarthritis that none of us can avoid, but allowing faulty curves and bony misalignments to persist may actually accelerate this degenerative process! Your Chiropractor may have you lie on a tightly rolled up towel (a frozen water bottle often feels even better) placed behind the neck and when it's comfortable, performing this on the edge of the bed is a great way to re-educate a reversed cervical curve (and, it feels GREAT!). Even a heel lift in the shoe of a short leg can help the neck! Spinal manipulation, manual mobilization techniques, and trained exercises all address this treatment goal quite effectively!

We will continue this conversation next month discussing the third and fourth topics: 3) Functional Restoration; and 4) Maintenance / Prevention, so STAY TUNED

Neck Pain Relief
The Most Important Factor

What every neck pain sufferer should know before choosing a doctor or starting any back pain treatment

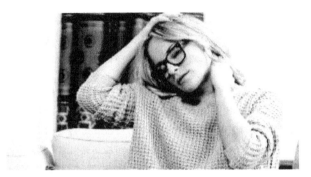

Lacey / Olympia – There is no doubt. Neck pain is can be life changing. Nothing is worse than being in constant pain – and not being able to do all the things you once could. And just as bad as the pain is the frustration of not being able to find a solution.

How would you like to finally find a solution for your neck pain? A solution that is 100% guaranteed to work and cure your neck pain… instantly?

The bad news is – there is no "100% guaranteed cure" for neck pain. And no ethical doctor would make such a claim. Real, ethical doctors use scientific research and do not make ridiculous claims. In other words, they are honest and up front with patients and give them the best options possible and are honest about the possible outcomes.

The good news is – there are some wonderful treatments for neck pain that often get great results. And because no one treatment works for everyone – the key is to find what treatment is right for your individual case.

That can be the difference between finally relieving your pain and continuing to suffer.

That's why the most important factor in finding relief for your neck pain is choosing the right doctor. That may seem obvious – but it is not what you think. Here is why...

It is very important to find a doctor that is "mainstream." This means they are knowledgeable about treatments that are scientifically based. It also means that they are well respected by their colleagues and actively refer to other doctors.

The most important thing is the doctor you choose should be "patient centered." This means he or she always finds out what you want – and gives it to you.

Because this is so important a large group of Chiropractic Physicians Doctors of Chiropractic who have joined forces and taken an amazing pledge in an effort to let patients know what kind of care you can expect.

These doctors are members of ChiroTrust and here is their pledge: **"To the best of my ability, I agree to provide my patients convenient, affordable, and mainstream Chiropractic care. I will not use unnecessary long-term treatment plans and/or therapies."**

In other words, if you choose a ChiroTrust doctor you can expect to get the best possible care and the doctor will try to get you better as soon as possible and out of the office.

In fact, ChiroTrust doctors do not offer multiple visit plans and will see you one visit at a time. Patients usually breathe a big sigh of relief because there is no long term commitment and they get to try out treatments and see if they like them.

And just as important – this makes treatment very affordable for patients without insurance coverage.

Here is something you need to know: ChiroTrust doctors do not just treat you by themselves in isolation. They have great relationships with other doctors in the community and will work with them to get you the best possible care for you individual case.

In other words, you will be going to a trusted advisor who will help you get exactly what you want.

If this sounds great and you would like to see if a ChiroTrust doctor can help you with your neck pain – you are going to love this...

160

Dr. David Warwick D.C. is a ChiroTrust doctor and his practice is at 8650 Martin Way East #207 right here in Lacey. He offers a limited amount of free consultations every month and if you would like one just call **360-951-4504**. Consultations are limited due to time constraints because Dr. Warwick always makes sure he has the time necessary for each and every patient. At the consultation you will get all your questions answered and given the best plan to help your neck pain. Of course, there is no obligation and it is completely free. If you are looking for more information provide your contact information below or visit our website DrDavidWarwick.com

Chiropractic Management of Neck Pain (Part 2)

Last month, we covered the first two of four primary goals when it comes to the chiropractic management of neck pain (#1 – Pain Management and #2 – Structural realignment). This month, we will conclude this discussion with #3 – Functional Restoration and #4 – Prevention.

3) FUNCTIONAL RESTORATION: Restoring function basically allows the patient to return to their pre-injury activities of daily living, which is the ultimate goal when managing all conditions! In order for this to happen, it is necessary to have the first two goals accomplished, and

the primary "tool" that we use to accomplish this goal is exercise training. There are several options to determine which exercise is most needed. A physical performance test can be done, which consists of a series of exercise-like maneuvers that we measure with an instrument that measures degrees (for range of motion), count repetitions (when testing for strength), or count time – usually in seconds (when testing for endurance, balance, and aerobic capacity). We then can compare you to the "norms" that have been published to see if you need help in a particular area. This also establishes a "baseline" or starting point to compare a month later after you've performed the proper exercises designed to improve that "failed test." The three primary goals of exercises include stretching, strengthening, and restoring coordination.

STRETCH: A very effective exercise is performed by bending the head to the right, reaching over with the right hand, and gently pulling on the head until a good stretch is felt on the left side of the neck. Reaching down with the opposite (left) arm (as if there's a dollar bill on the ground and you just can't quite reach it) enhances the stretch. While stretching, tuck in your chin, drop your head forwards and backwards, and turn your head a little from side to side to feel for different tight muscle fibers. Continue this stretch for 10-20 seconds or long enough to feel that you've accomplished a good stretch. Then, repeat this on the opposite side. This can be done sitting or standing, and most importantly, do this multiple times a day, especially when you feel tight – like at work, for example. There are other stretches but this actually combines four different exercises into one, so it's often enough!

STRENGTHENING: Place your hand against the side of your head and push your head into your hand using about 10-20% maximum effort (not much pressure!). First, allow your head "to win" by moving your head further until a tight stretch is felt. Second, let your hand "win" by moving the head to the opposite direction while maintaining pressure against your hand. Allow the head to bend ALL THE WAY to the end-range and repeat three times in each direction.

COORDINATION: Motor control, balance, and coordination are further enhanced by balancing on one foot with eyes open AND closed. Stand near a wall to avoid falling!

4. PREVENTION: Keep exercising and eat right! Consider joining a health club, working out with a friend, riding a bike, walking, and/or swimming. You choose!

Neck Pain – Drugs or Chiropractic?

When you have neck pain, do you instinctively reach for that bottle of ibuprofen or Tylenol? If so, is that the best option? Who can we trust for the answer? Since between 10-20% of the population suffer from chronic or persistent neck pain, this is a VERY IMPORTANT question!

If we look at the literature published in peer reviewed journals by authors who have no financial incentives in the outcome of the study, we can find accurate, non-biased information to answer this question. So, let's start with a landmark study published in SPINE, a leading medical journal that reviewed ALL the publications printed between 2000 and 2010 on neck pain – a total of 32,000 articles with over 25,000 hours of review. (Haldeman S, Carroll L, Cassidy JD, et. al. The Bone and Joint Decade 2000-2010 Task Force on Neck Pain and Its Associated Disorders: Executive Summary. Spine 2008,33(4S):S5-S7). This resulted in a 220 page comprehensive report from a multidisciplinary International Task Force involving seven years of work from 50+ researchers from 19 different clinical scientific disciplines worldwide looking at the MOST EFFECTIVE approaches available (both surgical and non-surgical) for patients suffering from neck pain.

Highlights from the study include the following:

1) Manipulation/mobilization are safe, effective, and appropriate treatment approaches for most patients with disabling neck pain (both traumatic and non-traumatic).

2) Neck pain patients should be informed of ALL effective treatment options so they can choose effectively.

3) The very rare risk of vertebrobasilar artery (VBI) stroke is NO DIFFERENT when comparing patients consulting a doctor of chiropractic verses a primary care medical physician as the stroke event, in most cases, has occurred prior to the visit.

4) The treatment option(s) available should consider the potential side effects and personal preferences of the patient.

5) For most neck pain patients, treatments that were found to be safe and effective include manipulation, mobilization, exercise, education, acupuncture, analgesics, massage, and low-level laser therapy.

6) For non-neurological neck pain, ineffective treatments (poor choices) include surgery, collars, TENS (transcutaneous electrical nerve stimulation), most injection therapies (including corticosteroid injections and rhizotomy).

7) For neck pain WITH nerve compression, there is very little research published on non-surgical care. Here, in the absence of serious pathology or progressive neurological loss, start with the most conservative (like chiropractic!) followed by more invasive treatments like epidural steroid injections (ESI's) and surgery.

8) Whiplash patients should follow similar guidelines as described above.

9) Some benefit from the chosen treatment should be seen within the first two to four weeks of care.

10) Be realistic about treatment goals – neck pain is often recurrent (comes and goes) as most people (50-80%) will NOT experience complete resolution of symptoms and will have neck pain again one to five years later.

Another study published in The Annals of Internal Medicine ("Spinal Manipulation, Medication, or Home Exercise with Advice for Acute and Subacute Neck Pain: A Randomized Trial. 3 January 2012, Vol.156, No. 1, Part 1) reports similar information favoring spinal manipulation and exercise, as these were found to be SUPERIOR to medication use. Another study reported excellent results for 27 patients utilizing chiropractic care who had herniated cervical disks WITH spinal cord compression verified on MRI (70% improved after an average of 12 visits)! TRY CHIROPRACTIC FIRST!!!

Chiropractic & Exercise vs. OTC Medication for Neck Pain?

"Boy, my neck is killing me! Honey, where is the ibuprofen?" Isn't this the FIRST thing people think of when they have an ache or pain? The general public does NOT usually think, "….boy, do I need to see my chiropractor – my neck is killing me!" So, the question of the month is, which one is better, chiropractic or over-the-counter (OTC) medication? Let's take a look.

Though this question has been discussed for years (just search: "chiropractic vs. NSAIDs"), a recent study looked specifically at this question, which will be the main focus of this Health Update. The study points out that it has been estimated that 75% of Americans will experience **neck pain** at some point in their life. For years, spinal manipulation has been criticized as being ineffective or providing limited benefits. Meanwhile, ads on TV, in magazines, and almost everywhere you look, show someone reaching for aspirin, ibuprofen, or even narcotics to manage their pain.

However, this new research clearly supports that seeing a chiropractor and/or engaging in light exercise can bring neck pain relief more effectively than relying on pain medications! Researchers even found that the benefits of chiropractic adjustments were still favored A YEAR LATER when comparing the differences between the spinal manipulation and medication treated groups! Moderate acute neck pain is one of the most frequent complaints prompting appointments at primary care/medical clinics and is estimated to account for millions of doctor visits per year. In some cases, pain and stiffness occurs without a known cause and there is no "standard" medical treatment. Though physical therapy, pain medication, and chiropractic have all been utilized for neck pain, until now no one had compared the benefits of each in a single study.

The study consisted of 272 neck pain subjects split up into three groups: 1) Chiropractic group (approximately 20-minute treatments an average of 15 times); 2) Pain medication group (meds included acetaminophen, and in some cases stronger prescription meds including narcotics and muscle relaxants); 3) Physical Therapy group (consisting of meeting twice and receiving advice and exercise instruction at 5-10 repetitions up to eight times a day).

At the end of three months, the chiropractic and exercise group did significantly better than those who took drugs. Approximately 57% of those receiving chiropractic management and 48% of those who did the exercises reported at least 75% reduction in pain vs. 33% of people in the medication group. A year after the treatment period ended, the numbers decreased to 53% in the chiropractic and exercise groups, compared to 38% in pain medication group. The chiropractic group received the highest scores in patient satisfaction at all time points. An interesting downside noted in the medication study group was that the subjects had to use a progressively greater amount of medication at a progressively increased frequency to manage their pain. Stomach trouble is the most common side effect of NSAIDs (leading to ulcers) as well as liver and kidney problems. Another interesting finding was that the subjects in the medication treated group felt less empowered, less active, and less in control over their own condition compared with those in the other two groups.

This study points out the benefits of two treatment approaches that chiropractors commonly utilize: spinal manipulation and exercise training/advice!

Neck Pain and Cervical Disk Herniation

Neck pain can arise from many sources. There are ligaments that hold bones to other bones that are non-elastic and very strong. When injured, the term, "sprain" is applied. The muscle and/or its attachment (the tendon) can tear as well, which is called a "strain." But, what is it that people refer to when they say, "…I slipped a disk in my neck!"?

The disks lay between the vertebrae in the front of the spine, and they are part of the primary support and shock absorbing system of our neck and back. There are 6 disks in the neck, 12 in the mid-back and 5 in the low back for a total of 23. The disks in the low back are big, like the vertebral bodies they lie between, and get progressively smaller as they go up the spine towards the head. When we bend our neck forwards, the disk compresses, and opens wider when we look up. It forms a wedge shape when we side bend left or right, and it twists when we rotate or turn the head.

The terms, "...a slipped disk, a herniated disk, a ruptured disk, a bulging disk" (and more), all mean something similar, if not exactly the same thing. A central part of the disk is liquid-like and can herniate in any direction. When it does, it can create pain IF it pinches something, or it may be painless if it doesn't. In fact, since the invention of the CAT scan and MRI, many ("normal") people have been found on the scan to have some type of disk "derangement" (alteration of the normal integrity of the disk), with 50%+ showing bulging disk(s) and 21% showing frank herniations WITH NO PAIN AT ALL! So, in the absence of shooting pain down an arm from the neck, or when there is no numbness or weakness in the arm, why order an MRI? It may show bulges or herniations that are not "clinically" important, and may falsely lead a doctor to recommend surgery when it's not needed.

There are "KEY" findings in the history and examination that leads us to the diagnosis of a cervical disk injury. From the history, the disk patient often has arm pain, numbness, and/or muscle weakness that follows a specific pathway, such as numbness to the thumb/index finger (C6 nerve), middle of the hand & 3rd finger (C7) or to the pinky & ring finger (C8). Certain positions, such as looking up, usually irritate the neck and arm, and bending the head forward relieves it. Another unique history and exam finding is if the patient finds relief by putting the arm up and over their head. Similarly, letting the arm hang down is often associated with irritation. Other examination findings unique to a cervical disk injury include reproducing the arm pain by placing the head in certain positions such as bending the head back and to the side simultaneously. Another is compressing the head into the shoulders. When lifting up on the head (traction), relief of arm pain is common. The neurological exam will usually show a reduction of sensation when we gently poke them with a sharp object, and/or they may have weakness when compared to the opposite side.

Chiropractic treatments can be very successful in resolving cervical disk herniation signs and symptoms, and should CERTAINLY be tried before agreeing to a surgical correction. Often, the surgeon will recommend a fusion of 2 or more neck vertebrae, sometimes with a metal plate in the front of the spine. This increases the load on either side of the fusion and can create problems above and below the fusion. Trust me, try chiropractic first. You'll be glad you did!

Neck Pain Treatment Options

Neck pain is a very common problem. In fact, 2/3rds of the population will have neck pain at some point in life. It can arise from stress, lack of sleep, prolonged postures (such as reading or driving), sports injuries, whiplash injuries, arthritis, referred pain from upper back problems, or even from sinusitis! Rarely, it can be caused from dangerous problems including referred pain during a heart attack, carotid or vertebral artery injuries, or head or neck cancer, but these, as previously stated, are very uncommon. However, since you don't know why your neck hurts, it's very important to have your neck pain properly evaluated so the cause can be properly treated and not just covered up from the use of pain killers!

Barring the dangerous causes of neck pain listed above, treatment methods vary depending on whom you elect to consult. Classically, if you see your primary care physician, pharmaceutical care is usually the approach. Medications can be directed at reducing pain (Tylenol, or one of many prescription "pain killers"), at reducing inflammation and pain (Aspirin, Ibuprofen, Aleve, etc.), to reduce muscle spasms (like muscle relaxers) or, medications may be directed to reduce depression, anxiety, or the like. When a sinus infection affects the 2 deep sinuses (ethmoid and sphenoid sinuses which are located deep in the head), the referred pain is directed to the back of the head and neck. Here, an antibiotic may be needed and/or something specifically directed at allergies when present. In general, in cases that do not respond to usual chiropractic care, co-management with the primary care physician is a good option.

However, the good news is that chiropractic care usually works well, and the need for medication can be avoided since the side effects of medication can sometimes be worse than the benefits. Recently, The Bone and Joint Decade Task Force on Neck Pain published arguably the best review of research published between 2000 and 2010 regarding neck pain treatment approaches. They concluded that spinal manipulation and mobilization are highly effective for many causes of neck pain, especially when arising from the muscles and joints – the most common cause. Therefore it would seem logical to consult with a Chiropractor FIRST since manipulation and mobilization are so effective and safe. When we add neck exercises, the results are even better, according to some studies. As chiropractors, we will often use different modalities including electric stimulation, ultrasound, hot and/or cold (which are usually given as a good home-applied remedy), and others. In particular, low level laser therapy (LLLT) has been shown, "…to reduce pain immediately after treatment in acute neck pain and up to 22 weeks after completion of treatment in patients with chronic neck pain" [Lancet, 2009; 374(9705)]. LLLT is a commonly used modality by chiropractors and when combined with spinal manipulation, the results can be even faster! We will also evaluate your posture, body mechanics, and consider "ergonomic" or work station problems and offer recommendations for improving your work environment. We also frequently utilize anti-inflammatory nutrients including vitamins, minerals, herbs, and more to avoid the negative side effects to the stomach, liver, and kidney negative that can result from using non-steroidal anti-inflammatory drugs (NSAIDs) like aspirin, ibuprofen, or Aleve. Make chiropractic your FIRST choice when neck pain strikes, NOT last resort!

Neck Pain and Chiropractic

Neck pain represents a major problem for people throughout the world with considerable negative impact on individuals, families, communities, health care systems, and businesses. Up to 70% of the general population will have neck pain at some point in their life. Recovery within the year from neck pain ranges between 33% and 65%, AND relapses are common throughout the life time of the neck pain patient. Generally, neck pain is more common in women, higher in high-income countries, and higher in urban regions. The greatest risk of developing neck pain occurs between 35 and 49 years of age. Since neck pain, very similar to low back pain, is very common and likely to recur over and over again, the question is, what is the best course of action regarding treatment?

A recent study on neck pain patients compared the effectiveness of manual therapy performed by a chiropractor, physical therapy performed by a physical therapist (PT), and medical care performed by medical physician (MD). The success rate determined at the seventh week was TWO TIMES BETTER for the manual therapy/chiropractic group (68.3%) compared to the medical care group. Those receiving manual therapy also had fewer absences from work compared to both the medical and PT treated groups. Lastly, both the manual therapy and PT groups used less pain relief medication compared to the medically treated group. Another study looked at the multiple approaches that chiropractors use for treating patients with neck pain to determine the "best" approach a chiropractor can use. They reported 94% had improvement or less neck pain after just one treatment when the mid-back (thoracic spine) was also adjusted. Similarly, after receiving two treatments over a one week time frame, the group receiving midback adjustments (vs. the group who did not) reported lower pain and disability scores. A similar study concluded that the best results occurred when the neck, upper back/lower neck, and mid-back were adjusted. This group, when compared to neck adjustments alone, reported greater reductions in disability scores. Thus, having the cervical spine, upper back, and mid-back all adjusted appears to yield quicker, more satisfying results than neck adjustments alone.

What about the role of exercise in the management of neck pain patients? In November 2012, a systematic review of manual therapies for nonspecific neck pain reported that the addition of neck exercises to a treatment plan provided more benefits than spinal manipulation alone. Similarly, in September 2012 (The Annals of Internal Medicine), chiropractic adjustments were compared against exercise and pain medication treatment groups involving 272 patients tracked over a one-year time frame after a 12-week treatment. Both the chiropractic and exercise groups experienced the most significant pain reduction when compared to the medication treated group with more than double the likelihood of complete pain relief. The chiropractic and exercise groups also had the best short and long term results, but ONLY the chiropractic group found the benefits to last a year or more. The authors (Bronfort, et. al) reported the success of chiropractic treatment stems from its ability to address the CAUSE of the problem rather than simply addressing the symptoms!

How Many Lacey / Olympia Baby Boomers Get Neck Pain Relief...

Are Lacey / Olympia Residents In Their 50s and 60s Getting More Pain Relief Than Earlier Generations?

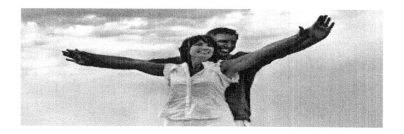

Lacey / Olympia – If you are in your 50s or 60s – you know this is true. Baby Boomers are different. Earlier generations accepted limitations and "settled." You always expected and got more. That's why when Baby Boomers hit their 50s or 60s and started getting more aches and pains – they searched for a solution that would allow them to get out of pain and continue their active lifestyles. Most importantly – they searched with an open mind this opened the door to many "alternative" treatments that were unjustly frowned upon not too long ago.

Here's something extremely important: Baby Boomers also questioned the way things had always been. They completely understand pain medications did do not always give them the relief they wanted – and can came come will with serious side effects. And everyone knows most know the risks associated with spine surgery. They wanted a treatment with two things – It worked and was natural.

As more and more Baby Boomers started trying natural options – more research was done. And as research started showing proof – open minded doctors started using the best less common treatments with great results. One treatment that many Baby Boomers flock to is, have embraced is "Spinal manipulative therapy" or SMT. That is a big word for a chiropractic adjustment. With an increase in research, SMT has finally been accepted in the medical community and gone mainstream. This means more pain relief for more neck pain sufferers. It's amazing how Baby Boomers were way ahead of this mainstream trend and have were always open and accepting of Chiropractors and their successful treatments long before it went mainstream.

Choosing A Chiropractor Are all Chiropractors the same? Just like anything – there are always good and bad… with varying degrees in between. That's why; the best way to find a great Chiropractor is by referral from someone you trust.

But here is one BIG factor you should think about when choosing… Many Chiropractors dictate care to patients – selling long term treatment plans. In other words, they some may want you to commit to months and months of care that can cost thousands of dollars. You must pay out of your own pocket. Others believe in a much more flexible approach. There is no commitment or expensive long term plans. They see patient's one visit at a time and let patients decide if it is something they want to continue or not. This also makes care very affordable.

This is the approach modern thinking Baby Boomers love and has caused them to flock to likeminded doctors' offices for neck pain treatment. What's amazing is hundreds of doctors around the country joined forces in a group called, "ChiroTrust." In an effort to let patents know exactly what to expect, they have actually taken this pledge and display it in their offices…**"To the best of my ability, I agree to provide my patients convenient, affordable, and mainstream Chiropractic care. I will not use unnecessary long-term treatment plans and/or therapies."** This pledge is proudly displayed in Dr. David Warwick's office located at 8650 Martin Way East #207 Lacey 98516.

For more information on Chiro-Trust, go to www.Chiro-Trust.org to find out more about the doctor. If you are suffering with neck pain and would like to see if Dr. Warwick can help you – just give he a call and he will give you a complimentary consultation. Like always – there is no further obligation – it is just a way to meet Dr. Warwick, get all your questions answered and find out if this

Neck Pain – Chiropractic and the Older Patient

People of all ages suffer from neck pain, and many frequently turn to chiropractors for care because it's been found to be one of the most effective and efficient forms of treatment available, and it carries minimal side effects! It has been projected that by 2030, nearly one in five US residents will be 65 or older. Currently, approximately 14% of the patients treated by chiropractors are 65 or older, making it one of the most frequently utilized forms of complementary and alternative care used by older adults. What kind of care can a senior citizen expect when seeking treatment from a chiropractor? Let's take a look!

Musculoskeletal pain, or pain in the neck, back, arms, and/or legs, drives the majority of elderly patients to chiropractors. While low back and neck pain are the most common complaints, it's not unusual for patients to also have one or two other conditions (or more) that they did NOT know chiropractic care could help. In fact, common "goals" for managing every patient (not just the elderly) include services related to patient assessment, maintenance of health, and prevention of illness, in addition to treatment of illness or injury. Common chiropractic treatment approaches include spinal manipulation and/or mobilization, nutritional counseling, physical activity/exercise, and (especially important for the elderly population) fall prevention.

We will now focus on neck pain as it relates to the elderly population and the various chiropractic management strategies that might be encountered by an elderly patient. Common reasons patients present regarding the neck include limited movement, stiffness, and pain. Neck pain can also interfere with sleep, as finding a comfortable position in bed can be quite challenging! Lifting, carrying, and playing with grandchildren is a very common issue for either causing a new complaint or irritating an existing one. Neck pain may also interfere with reaching and lifting. Thus, activities like yard or garden work may become more difficult and less enjoyable. Neck pain is often associated with headaches, which can make daily tasks even more challenging.

When an elderly patient visits a chiropractor for the first time or for a new complaint, he/she can expect to fill out some initial paperwork, as well as provide a history of the main complaint and any lesser complaints. This may also include providing a family and medical history. The examination usually includes general observations, palpating or feeling for muscle tightness, tenderness, warm/cool, range of spinal motion (neck, back, extremities), orthopedic tests, neurological tests, and possibly x-rays. Treatment of the neck may include massage or mobilization to loosen up the neck, manipulation to free up restricted joint motion, and even exercise training. The goal of treatment is to improve neck motion, activity tolerance, and quality of life (less pain, improved sleep, etc.). So, whether you are 10, 20, 50, 70, or 90 years old, give chiropractic a chance to help you manage your neck pain!

Neck Pain: Where Is It Coming From?

Neck pain can arise from a number of different tissues in the neck. Quite often, pain is generated from the small joints in the back of the vertebra (called facets). Pain can also arise from disk related conditions where the liquid-like center part of the disk works its way out through cracks and tears in the thicker outer part of the disk and can press on nerves producing numbness and/or weakness in the arm. It is possible to "sprain" the neck in car accidents, sports injuries, or from slips and falls. This is where ligaments tear and lose their stability resulting in excessive sliding back and forth of the vertebrae during neck movements. When muscles or their tendon attachments to bone are injured, these injuries are called "strains" and pain can occur wherever the muscle is torn. There is also referred pain. Here, the injury is at a distance away from where the pain is felt. A classic referred pain pattern is shoulder blade pain when a disk in the neck herniates. Let's take a closer look at two conditions we often diagnose and treat as chiropractors:

Spinal Stenosis: This occurs when the canals in the spine narrow to the point of pinching the spinal cord in the trefoil shaped central canal (called "central stenosis") or when the nerve roots get pinched in the lateral recesses (called lateral recess stenosis). This can occur from arthritis in the facet joints, disk bulging or herniations, thickening of ligaments, shifting of one vertebra over another, aging, heredity (being born with a narrowed canal), and/or from tumors. Usually, combinations of several of the above occur simultaneously. When this is present in the neck, it can be more serious compared to stenosis in the low back as the spinal cord ends at the upper part of the low back (T12 level) so only the nerves get pinched. Stenosis in the neck however pinches the spinal cord itself. Symptoms can include pain in one or both arms, but it's more dangerous when leg pain, numbness, or weakness occur (called myelopathy). Rarely, loss of bowel or bladder control can occur which is then considered a "medical emergency" and requires prompt surgery.

Cervical Disk Herniation: As previously stated, the liquid-like center of the disk can work its way through cracks and tears in the outer layer of the disk and press on a nerve resulting in numbness, pain, and/or weakness in the arm. The classic presentation is the patient finding relief by holding the arm over the head, as this puts slack in the nerve and it hurts less in this position. The position of the head also makes a difference as looking up usually hurts more and can increase the arm pain/numbness while looking down reduces the symptoms. We will carefully test your upper extremity neurological functions (reflexes, muscle strength, and sensation as each nerve performs a different function in the arm), and we can tell you which nerve is pinched after a careful examination. This condition can lead to surgery so please take this seriously.

The good news is that chiropractic care can manage both spinal stenosis and cervical disk herniations BEFORE they

181

reach the point of requiring surgery. So make chiropractic your FIRST choice when neck pain occurs!

Neck Pain Treatment Options

Neck pain is a very common problem. In fact, 2/3rds of the population will have neck pain at some point in life. It can arise from stress, lack of sleep, prolonged postures (such as reading or driving), sports injuries, whiplash injuries, arthritis, referred pain from upper back problems, or even from sinusitis! Rarely, it can be caused from dangerous problems including referred pain during a heart attack, carotid or vertebral artery injuries, or head or neck cancer, but these, as previously stated, are very uncommon. However, since you don't know why your neck hurts, it's very important to have your neck pain properly evaluated so the cause can be properly treated and not just covered up from the use of pain killers!

Barring the dangerous causes of neck pain listed above, treatment methods vary depending on whom you elect to consult. Classically, if you see your primary care physician, pharmaceutical care is usually the approach. Medications can be directed at reducing pain (Tylenol, or one of many prescription "pain killers"), at reducing inflammation and pain (Aspirin, Ibuprofen, Aleve, etc.), to reduce muscle spasms (like muscle relaxers) or, medications may be directed to reduce depression, anxiety, or the like. When a sinus infection affects the 2 deep sinuses (ethmoid and sphenoid sinuses which are located deep in the head), the referred pain is directed to the back of the head and neck. Here, an antibiotic may be needed and/or something specifically directed at allergies when present. In general, in cases that do not respond to usual chiropractic care, co-management with the primary care physician is a good option.

However, the good news is that chiropractic care usually works well, and the need for medication can be avoided since the side effects of medication can sometimes be worse than the benefits. Recently, The Bone and Joint Decade Task Force on Neck Pain published arguably the best review of research published between 2000 and 2010 regarding neck pain treatment approaches. They concluded that spinal manipulation and mobilization are highly effective for many causes of neck pain, especially when arising from the muscles and joints – the most common cause. Therefore it would seem logical to consult with a Chiropractor FIRST since manipulation and mobilization are so effective and safe. When we add neck exercises, the results are even better, according to some studies. As chiropractors, we will often use different modalities including electric stimulation, ultrasound, hot and/or cold (which are usually given as a good home-applied remedy), and others. In particular, low level laser therapy (LLLT) has been shown, "…to reduce pain immediately after treatment in acute neck pain and up to 22 weeks after completion of treatment in patients with chronic neck pain" [Lancet, 2009; 374(9705)]. LLLT is a commonly used modality by chiropractors and when combined with spinal manipulation, the results can be even faster! We will also evaluate your posture, body mechanics, and consider "ergonomic" or work station problems and offer recommendations for improving your work environment. We also frequently utilize anti-inflammatory nutrients including vitamins, minerals, herbs, and more to avoid the negative side effects to the stomach, liver, and kidney negative that can result from using non-steroidal anti-inflammatory drugs (NSAIDs) like aspirin, ibuprofen, or Aleve. Make chiropractic your FIRST choice when neck pain strikes, NOT last resort!

Neck Pain and Cervical Disk Herniation

Neck pain can arise from many sources. There are ligaments that hold bones to other bones that are non-elastic and very strong. When injured, the term, "sprain" is applied. The muscle and/or its attachment (the tendon) can tear as well, which is called a "strain." But, what is it that people refer to when they say, "…I slipped a disk in my neck!"?

The disks lay between the vertebrae in the front of the spine, and they are part of the primary support and shock absorbing system of our neck and back. There are 6 disks in the neck, 12 in the mid-back and 5 in the low back for a total of 23. The disks in the low back are big, like the vertebral bodies they lie between, and get progressively smaller as they go up the spine towards the head. When we bend our neck forwards, the disk compresses, and opens wider when we look up. It forms a wedge shape when we side bend left or right, and it twists when we rotate or turn the head.

The terms, "…a slipped disk, a herniated disk, a ruptured disk, a bulging disk" (and more), all mean something similar, if not exactly the same thing. A central part of the disk is liquid-like and can herniate in any direction. When it does, it can create pain IF it pinches something, or it may be painless if it doesn't. In fact, since the invention of the CAT scan and MRI, many ("normal") people have been found on the scan to have some type of disk "derangement" (alteration of the normal integrity of the disk), with 50%+ showing bulging disk(s) and 21% showing frank herniations WITH NO PAIN AT ALL! So, in the absence of shooting pain down an arm from the neck, or when there is no numbness or weakness in the arm, why order an MRI? It may show bulges or herniations that are not "clinically" important, and may falsely lead a doctor to recommend surgery when it's not needed.

There are "KEY" findings in the history and examination that leads us to the diagnosis of a cervical disk injury. From the history, the disk patient often has arm pain, numbness, and/or muscle weakness that follows a specific pathway, such as numbness to the thumb/index finger (C6 nerve), middle of the hand & 3rd finger (C7) or to the pinky & ring finger (C8). Certain positions, such as looking up, usually irritate the neck and arm, and bending the head forward relieves it. Another unique history and exam finding is if the patient finds relief by putting the arm up and over their head. Similarly, letting the arm hang down is often associated with irritation. Other examination findings unique to a cervical disk injury include reproducing the arm pain by placing the head in certain positions such as bending the head back and to the side simultaneously. Another is compressing the head into the shoulders. When lifting up on the head (traction), relief of arm pain is common. The neurological exam will usually show a reduction of sensation when we gently poke them with a sharp object, and/or they may have weakness when compared to the opposite side.

Chiropractic treatments can be very successful in resolving cervical disk herniation signs and symptoms, and should CERTAINLY be tried before agreeing to a surgical correction. Often, the surgeon will recommend a fusion of 2 or more neck vertebrae, sometimes with a metal plate in the front of the spine. This increases the load on either side of the fusion and can create problems above and below the fusion. Trust me, try chiropractic first. You'll be glad you did!

Common Questions about Cervical Disk Herniations

Last month, we discussed the topic of **neck pain** arising from cervical disk herniations. The focus of this month's Health Update is common questions that arise from patients suffering from cervical disk derangement.

1. "What can I do to help myself for my herniated disk in my neck?" The mnemonic device "PRICE" stands for P rotect, R est, I ce C ompress, and E levate is a good tool to use in the acute stage of many musculoskeletal conditions.

- Protect your health by NOT placing yourself in an environment that is likely to harm you, such as playing sports or doing heavy yard work. That is, think about what you do BEFORE you do it and if sharp, radiating pain occurs, STOP and assess the importance of what you are doing. Use the concept, "…don't pick at your cut." This means if you want the injury to heal, don't keep irritating it!
- Rest is similar. Limit your activities to those that can be done without increasing symptoms, especially radiating pain.
- Ice – The use of ice reduces swelling/inflammation, which reduces pain and promotes healing. Alternate it every 15-20 minutes (on/off/on/off/on) several times a day. You can also use contrast therapy (Ice/heat/ice/heat/ice) at 10/5/10/5/10 minute intervals to "pump" out the swelling.
- Compress – The use of a collar worn backwards, if it's more comfortable that way, can literally "take the load off." the neck and disks. There are even inflatable collars which are pumped up with air to traction the neck. Other forms of traction will be discussed further.
- Elevate – The concept of raising the ankle to the height of the heart so swelling can drain out of the ankle is the classic example of "elevation." In the neck, the traction concept may apply once again.

2. "I don't want to have surgery if I can help it. What can you do as a chiropractor to help me?" This is one of our primary goals, and in fact, the goal of ALL health care providers, even surgeons! Chiropractic offers anti-inflammatory measures: ice, herbal anti-inflammatory agents (ginger, turmeric, bioflavonoid, curcumin, bromelain, Rosemary extract, Boswellia Extract, and more), digestive enzymes taken between meals, muscle relaxant nutrients (valerian root, vitamin D, a B complex,

chamomile, magnesium, and others) as well as other non-pharmaceutical options. Treatments consist of manual manipulation, mobilization, traction (for home and office), modalities such as laser and low-level laser, electrical stimulation, magnetic field, ultrasound, and others. Most important is having a "coach" guide you through the stages of healing by first addressing the acute inflammatory stage (first 72 hrs.), the proliferative or reparative phase (up to 6-8 weeks), followed by the remodeling phase (8 weeks to 1 or 2 years) and finally, the contraction phase (lifetime – includes the natural shortening of scar tissue). If manual traction reduces neck and arm pain, the use of home traction is very effective. Options include sitting over-the-door traction, laying down versions, and mobile traction collars (discussed previously). Exercises to stretch and strengthen the neck are also very important in reducing neck pain as well as preventing recurrences. If in spite of all the best efforts of this non-surgical care approach should ongoing neurological loss and relentless symptoms continue, we will coordinate care with physiatrists for possible injection therapy and pharmaceuticals, with neurology for further testing (such as EMG/NCV – a nerve test), and/or neuro- or orthopedic surgery – THE LAST RESORT!

Best Treatment For Neck Pain?

Research is helping doctors understand and treat neck pain – what you should know

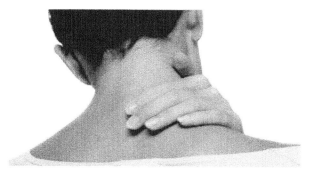

Lacey / Olympia WA – Neck pain is horrible. It can be impossible to find a position that does not hurt. Nothing is more frustrating than sleepless night after sleepless night turning you into an exhausted zombie.

But the most frustrating part is not knowing how to get relief.

Because about 70% of people suffer with neck pain at some point in their life – there is no shortage of, "wonder cures" on the market. Sadly, most of these products are better at getting money from you than they are at eliminating neck pain.

So here's a questions for you: Wouldn't it be nice to know what the best treatment for neck pain is? **And even better** – wouldn't it be a huge relief to know... for sure... you were doing the right thing to relieve your pain as fast as possible?

All that sounds wonderful – but here is some honest truth you should understand…

All cases of neck pain are individual. Therefore, there is no "one best treatment" for everyone. Honest and ethical doctors understand this and would never make such a claim.

But recent research has compared several treatments and one came out on top. If you suffer with neck pain… you will want to know this…

What's Better For Neck Pain…Medical Care, Physical Therapy Or Chiropractic?

A recent study on neck pain patients compared the effectiveness of manual therapy performed by a chiropractor, physical therapy performed by a physical therapist (PT), and medical care performed by medical physician (MD). The success rate determined at the seventh week was *TWO TIMES BETTER* for the manual therapy/chiropractic group (68.3%) compared to the medical care group.

Those receiving manual therapy also had fewer absences from work compared to both the medical and PT treated groups.

Lastly, both the manual therapy and PT groups used less pain relief medication compared to the medically treated group.

What's The Best Chiropractic Approach For Neck Pain?

Another study looked at the multiple approaches that chiropractors use for treating patients with neck pain to determine the "best" approach a chiropractor can use.

They reported 94% had improvement or less neck pain after just one treatment when the mid-back (thoracic spine) was also adjusted.

Similarly, after receiving two treatments over a one week time frame, the group receiving mid-back adjustments (vs. the group who did not) reported lower pain and disability scores.

A similar study concluded that the best results occurred when the neck, upper back/lower neck, and mid-back were adjusted. This group, when compared to neck adjustments alone, reported greater reductions in disability scores. Thus, having the cervical spine, upper back, and mid-back all adjusted appears to yield quicker, more satisfying results than neck adjustments alone.

Choosing A Chiropractor That Is Right For You

Just like all cases of neck pain are different – so are Chiropractors. And it is important to find one that is a good match for you.

One important thing to consider is if the doctor offers short term treatments that are affordable.

In other words, does the doctor treat you the least amount of times possible to get you out of pain – or do they sell long term plans that require a big commitment and a thousands of dollars.

Dr. David Warwick is a chiropractor in Lacey / Olympia WA who has seen his practice grow because he helps neck pain sufferers get out of pain with the least amount of treatments possible and without any long term commitment.

Patients love that he accepts them one visit at a time which give them the opportunity to see if they like the treatments and if they are working for them.

That's why Dr. Warwick offers a limited number of free consultations each month for neck pain sufferers.

These free consultations are a perfect opportunity to meet Dr. Warwick, get all your questions answered… and find out if he can help you.

Dr. Warwick is also a ChiroTrust member. (For more info., go to www.Chiro-Trust.org)

Does Neck Surgery Improve Long Term Outcomes?

How many times have you heard, "I have a pinched nerve in my neck and have to have surgery." Though there certainly are cases where surgical intervention is required, surgery should ONLY be considered after ALL non-surgical treatment approaches have been tried first (and failed). It is alarming how many cases of cervical radiculopathy (i.e., "pinched nerve") end up being surgically treated with NO trial of non-surgical care. Hence, the focus of this month's article will look at research ("MEDICAL EVIDENCE") that clearly states neck surgery DOES NOT improve the long term outcomes of patients with chronic **neck pain**.

Chronic neck pain (CNP) is, by definition, neck pain that has been present for a minimum of three months. This category of neck pain is very well represented, as many neck pain sufferers have had neck pain, "…for years" or, at least longer than three months. Depending on the intensity of pain and its effect on daily function, many patients with CNP often ask their primary care provider, "…is there anything surgically that can be done?" The desire for a "quick fix" is often the focus of those suffering with neck pain. Unfortunately, according to recent studies, there may not be a "quick fix" or, at least surgery is NOT the answer. The December 2012 issue of The European Spine Journal reports that spine surgery did NOT improve outcomes for patients with CNP. Moreover, they pointed to other studies that showed some VERY STRONG REASONS NOT to have spine surgery unless everything else has failed. One of the reasons was a higher hospital readmission rate after spine surgery. Another reported that most studies on surgical vs. conservative [non-surgical] care showed a high risk of bias, suggesting the research on surgical intervention was biased in the research approach used. They further reported, "The benefit of surgery over conservative care is not clearly demonstrated." It is important to point out that the research analyzed studies that included patients with and without radiculopathy (radiating arm pain from a pinched nerve), and myelopathy (those with pinching of the spinal cord creating pain, numbness, weakness in the legs, and/or bowel / bladder dysfunction).

In February of 2008, the Neck Pain Task Force published overwhelming evidence that research supports the use of cervical spinal manipulation in the treatment of both acute and chronic neck pain with or without radiculopathy. Bronfort published similar findings in 2010 in a large UK based study that looked at the published evidence supporting different types of treatment for various conditions. They found cervical spine manipulation was effective for neck pain of ANY duration (acute or chronic). Chiropractic utilizes manipulation, manual traction, mobilization, muscle release techniques, home cervical traction, exercise, as well as a multitude of physiotherapy modalities when managing patients with CNP. Given the overwhelming research evidence that surgical intervention for CNP is NOT any better than non-surgical care, the greater amount of negative side-effects, and the obviously long recovery time post-surgically, chiropractic treatment of anyone suffering from CNP should be tried FIRST.

Cervical Traction – The Many Options and How To Use It!

Last month, we looked at the published evidence that overwhelmingly supports the use of cervical traction. As promised, this month's focus is the proper methods of applying it. The type of traction that this discussion will address will be limited to the kind that can be purchased and then used in the home, usually multiple times a day, giving it a clear advantage over in-office traction treatments which can only be applied a few times a week during office visits. In some cases however, it may be appropriate to use the in-office type for a few sessions to determine dosage and/or tolerance prior to administering a home unit, but this varies from case to case, and each type of traction unit is different. In the **neck** or cervical spine, there are many varieties including: sitting over-the-door types, cervical collar types, as well as supine (lying on the back) types. Each variety has its pros and cons and prices vary considerably from $10 to $600.

CONDITIONS: Probably the most common condition treated with cervical traction is "cervical radiculopathy," or a pinched nerve. When a nerve root in the neck is pinched, pain, numbness, tingling, and/or muscle weakness occurs in the area the particular nerve innervates. For example, if a patient presents with pain and numbness radiating down the arm to the thumb and index finger and/or have weakness in bending their elbow and extending their wrist, then we know that the C6 nerve is pinched. When pulling or stretching the neck relieves the arm pain, traction is usually helpful. If pain worsens, the person is probably not ready for traction yet.

PROTOCOL (DOSAGE): The key to a successful outcome using cervical traction is finding the right dosage. If you start with too much weight, it may leave you feeling sore, or worse, making you reluctant to try it a second time. Therefore, rather than relying on using a certain percentage of body weight, it's safest to start with less weight and then gradually increase it, such as 5# (# = pounds or .45 kg) for 15-20 minutes. If that dose feels fine, try 7#/15-20 min., then 9#, 11#, 13#, etc., until you find it just isn't quite as comfortable at the last weight. You have now found your current threshold and should drop down to the last most comfortable weight and use that for a few days and then MAYBE try increasing it again. Studies show a maximum stretch is usually achieved within 15-20 minutes, so extending the time longer may be less productive. Facing the over-the-door unit may be better tolerated than facing away. Try it both ways and you decide which feels best. The next most important issue is frequency.

How often to repeat the traction sessions depends on: 1. The condition's severity and your response; 2. Your time availability. If there is a severe nerve pinch with muscle twitching, weakness and dense numbness/tingling, then the traction be repeated MANY times a day, gradually increasing the weight to find the optimum amount. We've had people repeat the traction 10x/day! With the option of wearing a cervical collar traction unit, you can actually travel and/or do certain activities during traction. We've had people travel to and from work while performing traction! Since each case is unique, we'll discuss that individually. The bottom line, IT WORKS GREAT with proper chiropractic management and in many cases, surgery CAN be avoided!

Traction – Does It Help Neck Pain and Headaches?

Traction is defined as, "…the act of pulling a body part." Therefore, it is commonly used in many regions including legs, arms, low back, mid-back, and the neck. We will be limiting this discussion to cervical or neck traction, and the question of the month is, "…does it help patients with neck pain and headaches?" Though I'm assuming you already know, the answer is YES! You may want a little "proof," so here it goes!

1. REDUCES DISK PROTRUSIONS: In 2002, a medically based study found traction to be very effective in the treatment of cervical radiculopathies (pinched nerves in the neck that radiate pain into

the arms). A 2008 study using MRI (images) described the effect traction had on the disk protrusions in the neck reporting 25 of 35 (or 71%) were reduced while in traction with a 19% increase in the spacing (disk height) and improved neck range of motion after the traction was applied. They postulated that by pulling the vertebrae in the neck apart, there was a suction-like effect pulling the disk material back in place.

2. RECOMMENDED BY GUIDELINES: Around the world, guidelines have been published giving doctor's information that allows us to know how well certain forms of treatment work for different conditions. In a 2008 publication, it was reported that, "Clinicians should consider the use of mechanical intermittent cervical traction, combined with other interventions such as manual therapy and strengthening exercises, for reducing pain and disability in patients with neck and neck-related arm pain."

3. CLINICAL PREDICTION RULES: These help us determine who is most likely to benefit from a certain type of treatment (in this case cervical traction and exercise). If 3 of 5 variables are found, the likelihood of success with traction & exercise was reported to be 79%, and if 4 of the 5 are found, 90%. The 5 variables are: 1. Radiating neck to arm pain in certain positions; 2. Positive shoulder abduction sign; 3. Age >55years old; 4. Positive limb tension test; 5. Relief of symptoms using manual distraction test (if pain is relieved while the neck is being pulled).

4. INTERMITTENT AND CONTINUOUS TRACTION: Either way, significant improvement in neck and arm pain, neck mobility, and nerve function occurred with both approaches.

5. TRACTION VS. SURGERY: In this study, patients with radiating arm pain and positive neurological

findings on exam were offered a course of traction before surgical options. They reported 63 of 81, or 78%, of the patients experienced significant or total relief, 3 could not tolerate traction and 15 simply didn't respond. They concluded that when neck and arm symptoms with neurological deficits were present for 6 weeks, that 75% will respond to neck traction over the next 6 weeks.

There are MANY additional studies available that show well beyond doubt that cervical traction is a GREAT option in the management of **neck and arm pain** and sometimes headaches. Next time, we will discuss "HOW TO" apply cervical traction.

Is It My Neck or Thoracic Outlet Syndrome?

Neck pain can arise from many different sources, and the patient's clinical presentation can be quite similar making it a challenge to diagnose. One of those related, and sometimes co-existing conditions, is called thoracic outlet syndrome, or TOS. Let's first discuss the anatomy of the neck and the thoracic outlet so we all have a good "picture" in mind of what we're talking about.

TOS can arise from either blood vessel compression, nerve compression or both, making the ease of diagnosis difficult. Adding to the challenge, the "pinch" of the structure can occur at more than one place! The nerves and blood vessels can get pinched at the exiting holes in the spine ("neuroforamen"), by tight "scalene" muscles, under the collar bone (clavicle) and/or by a tight pectoralis minor muscle near the arm pit. Hence, the symptoms usually include pain and numbness in the shoulder, arm and hand (usually affecting the 4th & 5th fingers). It's our job to run different tests to figure out where the primary pinch or pinches are located so we can treat the right area.

The causes of TOS can be many, with one of the obvious being a fractured collar bone or clavicle. Another is from having an extra rib. As there is not a lot of room for an extra structure, this can be a point of compression for some (but doesn't create TOS in everyone). An overly tight scalene muscle, scar tissue, an extra-large muscle and so on can also result in pinching of the nerves and/or blood vessels.

Purses, backpacks, carrying golf clubs, a mailbag and the like can also cause a pinch. A seat belt injury in a car accident is yet another cause, either from the direct trauma, or later when scar tissue forms in the area.

Our posture alone (without trauma), such as a slouchy, slumped posture where the shoulders roll forwards can cause TOS and, large breasts and obesity also add to the list of risk factors. Women are affected 3x more than men. Certain jobs where reaching overhead or outwards such as waitresses, carpenters, electricians, increase TOS risk.

Neck Pain and Our Pillow!

The relationship between **neck pain** and our pillow is more important than most of us realize! Though we all may have at one time or another slept on a variety of surfaces, and used any number of pillows (flat, medium, bulky) made of different materials (foam, feather, air, water, or memory foam), it's usually not until neck pain and/or headaches start to become an issue that we start to think, "…how important is my pillow?" Thankfully, the question has been addressed in a randomized peer-reviewed study. So, what did they find out?

The goal of a pillow is to support the neck more so than the head. In a study headed by Dr. Liselott Persson, MD, of the department of neurosurgery at the University of Lund in Sweden, researchers tested whether specific neck pillows have any effect on neck pain, headache and sleep quality in people suffering with chronic (>3months), non-specific neck pain. They also researched whether there was an optimum or "best" type of pillow that was preferred by their 52 patient group. They used 4 different pillows, 1 "normal" pillow and 3 of which were specially designed, each having a different shape and consistency. Over a 4-10 week time frame, the pillows were randomly distributed to the neck pain group who then graded them according to comfort, the effects on neck pain, sleep quality and headache using a questionnaire, and also described the characteristics of an "ideal pillow." Researchers and participants concluded the "ideal pillow" (for reducing neck pain and headaches and improving quality of sleep) includes a soft pillow with good support under the neck's curve (lordosis).

There are many styles of contoured cervical or neck pillows that vary considerably. This study supports the use of a specially designed style over a normal pillow. So what are some of the things to look for? First, consider your neck's length and girth. When you look in a mirror, do you have a neck that is short vs. long or, narrow vs. wide? This will direct you to a pillow that has a larger "hump" for your neck to be cradled in if it's a long neck and, the height of the hump – taller for the slender neck or, shorter for the wide neck. Some pillows have 2 options of "hump" sizes (located on the long edges of the pillow) – one short and flat and the other side taller and wider. Others recommend lying in the middle of the pillow if you're a back sleeper vs. lying on the edge of pillow when sleeping on your sides. A measurement taken from the neck to the point of the shoulder determines if the pillow should be a small, medium, or large. Water filled and/or air filled pillows can be varied by the amount of water or air added. The bottom line of which is "best" is based on comfort and support. Regardless of which you choose, it can take several days to get used to the new pillow, so we recommend using the pillow for at least 1 week. By then, you'll know if you chose the right style

What Every Neck Pain Sufferer Should Know About Treatment Options

And Choosing A Doctor That Is Right For You

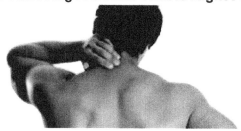

Lacey / Olympia WA – If you suffer with neck pain, you have probably already been to many doctors and tried several treatments... without great results.

Or maybe your neck pain is new and you don't know who to listen to. There are so many different treatments and "opinions," it can be extremely frustrating.

Even worse, if you have been told you have a herniated disc – the pain can be excruciating and the thought of facing back surgery can be terrifying.

What Are The Best Options?

Thankfully, research has been done that helps solve some of this puzzle – and give you some of the answers you are looking for. And now research has shown one treatment to be both safe and effective for many cases of neck pain.

But before we talk about this treatment – please understand this...

203

What you are about to discover is a REAL treatments performed by qualified doctors. This is NOT some "wonder cure" you see on Facebook or late night TV.

Here is the important truth: There is no 100% guaranteed cure for neck pain. No ethical doctor would ever guarantee results or lead you to believe they have a 100% cure for neck pain.

But there is a treatment that has already helped countless neck pain sufferers... possibly just like you.

In fact, The Bone and Joint Decade Task Force on Neck Pain published arguably the best review of research published between 2000 and 2010 regarding neck pain treatment approaches.

They concluded that this treatment is highly effective for many causes of neck pain, especially when arising from the muscles and joints – the most common cause.

We will get into more proof in just a minute but... but here is something you should know first... because the treatment is only as good as the doctor you choose...

There is a doctor using this treatment that has taken a very refreshing pledge that has led to neck pain sufferers flocking to his office.

This doctor's name is Dr. David Warwick and he is a Chiropractor in Lacey WA.

Here Is Something Extremely Important

You may have already been to a Chiropractor or just heard some things you did not like. So...
Why is this Chiropractor different and why are so many neck pain sufferers willing to give him a try – even when they have been to many other doctors already?

The answer is simple... Dr. Warwick took this pledge...

"To the best of my ability, I agree to provide my patients convenient, affordable, and mainstream Chiropractic care. I will not use unnecessary long-term treatment plans and/or therapies."
In other words, Dr. Warwick uses treatments that are widely accepted and has a goal to treat patients the least amount of times possible. He wants you feeling great and out of his office as soon as possible.

For this reason, Dr. Warwick NEVER tries to sell you a multiple visit, offers long term treatment plan that can cost thousands of dollars & multi-month treatment plans at a time.

Instead, Dr. Warwick does something his patients absolutely love – he accepts patients on a visit-by-visit basis. In other words, he treats you once and you decide if it is something you like and want to continue. There is no commitment and seeing patients as little as possible has made care extremely affordable – even if you do not have insurance coverage.

This no pressure, patient first approach it so refreshing, it has patients rant and raving… and the referrals have come in droves.

There is also one other thing about Dr. Warwick patients love…

Because he is mainstream, he works hand-in-hand with his colleagues in the medical community. Dr. Warwick gives and receives referrals from medical doctors all the time because his only goal is to give the patient (you) exactly what you want and is best for you.

What Is The Treatment And Is There Any Proof?

The treatment is spinal manipulation and mobilization-combined with exercise… and if you have neck pain – you are going to love this…

New research clearly supports that seeing a chiropractor and/or engaging in light exercise can bring neck pain relief more effectively than relying on pain medications! Researchers even found that the benefits of chiropractic adjustments were still favored A YEAR LATER when comparing the differences between the spinal manipulation and medication treated groups!

The study consisted of 272 neck pain subjects split up into three groups: 1) Chiropractic group (approximately 20-minute treatments an average of 15 times); 2) Pain medication group (meds included acetaminophen, and in some cases stronger prescription meds including narcotics and muscle relaxants); 3) Physical Therapy group (consisting of meeting twice and receiving advice and exercise instruction at 5-10 repetitions up to eight times a day).

At the end of three months, the chiropractic and exercise group did significantly better than those who took drugs. Approximately 57% of those receiving chiropractic management and 48% of those who did the exercises reported at least 75% reduction in pain vs. 33% of people in the medication group. A year after the treatment period ended, the numbers decreased to 53% in the chiropractic and exercise groups, compared to 38% in pain medication group. The chiropractic group received the highest scores in patient satisfaction at all time points.

Dr. Warwick is always 100% honest and he would like you to know this: Research helps doctors help patients – but no one should expect the results from this study or any other study. All patients are different and all cases are individual. That's why treatment outcomes can never be predicted for any one person. That is also why Dr. Warwick offers treatment with no long term commitment – so you can give it a try and see if it works for you.

Who Should Try This Treatment With Dr. Warwick?
You are may be a good candidate from this treatment if you have neck pain that originates from muscles or joints. If you are not sure, the best way to know if you are a candidate is to have a consultation with a qualified Chiropractic Physician.

Dr. Warwick's Invitation To You
Dr. Warwick is a ChiroTrust member (www.Chiro-Trust.org and offers a limited number of complimentary consultations every month. The purpose is to see if you are a good candidate for this treatment... and so you can get your questions answered. If you would like a complimentary consultation with Dr. Warwick, just call **360-951-4504** or DrDavidWarwick.com for more information. The best thing about the consultation is you will feel relieved finally getting some straight answers about your neck pain and what the best course of action is.

Neck and Headache Pain and Posture

Neck pain is one of the most common complaints for which patients present to chiropractic offices. Headaches are also another very common problem and often go hand-in-hand with the presence of neck pain. So, the question that is frequently asked is, "…why do headaches and neck pain often travel together?"

There are many types of headaches, some of which we have discussed previously with migraine and tension-type headaches being the most common. This month, the focus is on how headaches and the neck are related to each other and what YOU can do about it.

The relationship between neck pain and headaches is strong! In fact, in some cases, headaches will occur ONLY when the neck hurts. One reason is because the first three nerves that exit out from the top of the cervical spine (C1, 2 and 3) have to travel through the thick group of muscles that insert onto the back/base of the skull along the occipital rim. Because we carry a lot of stress in the neck muscles, when they tighten up, they squeeze or pinch those 3 nerves and pain then radiates into the back of the head and sometimes up and over the vertex to the eyes or behind the eyes. If you take your fingers or thumb and push firmly into those muscles at the very top of the neck or base of the skull, it often feels, "…like a good hurt." This is because they are usually tight since most of us carry our head too far forwards and the muscles have to contract and constantly work to keep the head from gliding even further.

So, what can YOU do about it? Let's talk about a few GREAT posture retraining exercises. Tuck in your chin to the point where the voice changes pitch (your voice will start to sound "funny"). At that point, release the chin slightly so the voice clears and stay in position! That is the posture or head position of choice. Initially, it will be very difficult to remember to hold that position very long because your muscles (and brain) aren't used to it and, you'll slip back into the old forward head carriage habit or chin poke position. So, be patient with yourself because it takes about 3 months of constant self-reminding to, "...keep that chin tucked," before this new "habit pattern" is formed in the brain.

Another great exercise is an "offshoot" of this, where you tuck the chin in as far as you can (making a double or triple chin) holding that position for 3 seconds, and then tip the head back as far as you can without releasing the chin tuck and hold for another 3 seconds. Repeat this 2-3x / "set" and perform this multiple times per day.

A 3rd great exercise for improving the forward head carriage posture is performed by lying on your back on a bed so that the edge of the bed is at the middle of the neck and head is dangling off the bed. Take a tightly rolled up towel (a hand size towel works well) and place it under the neck so that is resting on the edge of the bed so that your head can fall back towards the floor. Take some deep breaths and concentrate on relaxing all your neck muscles. Periodically, slowly rotate your head left to right, right to left, and "feel" the different muscles stretch as you do this. If you can afford 15 minutes, that's PERFECT! But, if you only have a few minutes it's still GREAT!

Between maintaining a chin tuck upright posture and retraining the curve in your neck with the head hang off the bed exercise, you'll feel (and look) much better!

Neck Pain: Manipulation vs. Other Treatments?

Mechanical **neck pain** affects an estimated 70% of people at some point in their lives. Many different treatment approaches are available for neck pain, making it very difficult for those suffering from neck pain to know which treatment approach(es) to choose. Research in this topic has revealed some very interesting information that places chiropractic and spinal manipulation in a VERY STRONG POSITION – in fact, at the TOP OF THE HEAP!

One such study looked at benefits of spinal manipulative therapy (SMT) in patients with acute and subacute neck pain. This study compared three study groups: 1. SMT only, 2. medication only, and 3. Home exercise and advice (HEA). This study randomized 272 neck pain patients suffering from neck pain for 2 to 12 weeks into a 12 week treatment period using 1 of the 3 treatment approaches tracking the results with the participant-rated pain as the primary treatment outcome measure. Secondary outcome data was obtained from other approaches. The results showed that the group treated with SMT, "...had a statistically significant advantage over medication after 8, 12, 26 and 52 weeks. HEA also had a statistical advantage over medication. Lastly, similar benefits were calculated between the SMT and exercise group. The conclusions support SMT and exercise/advise to be the choice over medication for acute and subacute neck pain patients. Regarding exercise, a similar study showed that "high-dosed supervised strengthening exercise" with and without SMT, was superior to a "low dose home mobilization exercise and advice group at 4, 12, 26, and 52 weeks."

211

Regarding chronic neck pain patients (that means pain that has been present for greater than 3 months), this study evaluated the changes that occurred in 191 patients. These patients were randomized to 11 weeks of 1 of 3 treatment groups and evaluated at 3, 6, 12, & 24 months after treatment. The 3 treatment options included: 1. Spinal manipulative therapy (SMT) only, 2. SMT with low-tech neck exercises, or, 3. A form of exercise using a MedX rehab machine. The results support the highest level of patient satisfaction was found in the 2nd group (SMT with low-tech exercise), suggesting that when patients present for treatment, spinal manipulation with low-tech exercises results in the most satisfied patient. These findings are important as this study evaluated the LONG-TERM benefits in patients who have had neck pain for a long time (i.e., "chronic"), where most studies only look at the short-term benefits.

Similar conclusions were reported from perhaps the largest scale study on neck pain based on research from 1980 to 2006 on the use, effectiveness and safety of noninvasive treatment approaches for neck pain and associated disorders. Their review of over 350 articles supported manual therapy (manipulation and mobilization) and supervised exercise to again, SHINE in their conclusions.

What is important is that ALL these studies support what chiropractors do: manipulate the neck and give supervised exercises! So, what are you waiting for? SPREAD THE WORD to everyone that you know who has neck pain – CHIROPRACTIC MAY BE THE BEST CHOICE!!!

The Neck and Headache Connection

When we hear the term headache, we don't usually think about the neck. Rather, we focus on the head, more specifically, "…what part of the head hurts?" But, upon careful questioning of patients, we usually find some connection or correlation between **neck pain** and headaches.

The key to this connection can be found in looking at the anatomy of the neck. There are 7 vertebrae that make up the cervical spine and 8 sets of nerves that exit this part of the spine and innervate various parts of the head, neck, shoulders and arms, all the way to the fingers. Think of the nerves as electric wires that stretch between a switch and a light bulb. When you flip on the switch, the light illuminates. Each nerve, as it exits the spine, is like a switch and the target it travels to represents the light bulb. So, if one were to stimulate each of the nerves as they exit the spine, we could "map" exactly where each nerve travels (of course, this has been done). When we look specifically at the upper 3 sets of nerves that exit the spine (C1, C2, and C3), we see that as soon as they exit the spine, they immediately travel upwards into the head (the scalp). Like any nerve, if enough pressure is applied to the nerve, some alteration in nerve function occurs and usually a sensory change is noted (numbness, tingling, pain, burning, etc.). If the pressure continues, these symptoms can last for a long time. These types of headaches are often called "cervicogenic headaches" (literally meaning headaches that are caused by the neck). These can be caused by the nerves getting pinched by tight muscles through which they travel as they make their way to the scalp.

Another connection between the neck and headaches includes the relationship between 2 of the 12 cranial nerves and the first three nerves in the neck described above. These types of headaches usually only affect one half of the head – the left or right side. One of the cranial nerves is called the trigeminal nerve (cranial nerve V). Because the trigeminal nerve innervates parts of the face and head, pain can also involve the face. Another cranial nerve (spinal accessory, cranial nerve IX) can also interact with the upper 3 cervical nerve roots, resulting in cervicogenic headaches. People with cervicogenic headaches will often present with an altered neck posture, restricted neck movement, and pain when pressure is applied to the base of the skull or to the upper vertebrae. Other than a possible numbness, there are no clinical tests that we can run to "show" this condition, though some patients may report scalp numbness or, it may be found during examination.

Though medication, injections, and even surgical options exist, manipulation applied to the small joints of the neck, especially in the upper part where C1-3 exit, works really well so why not try that first as it's the least invasive and, VERY EFFECTIVE! In some cases, a combination of approaches may be needed but many times, chiropractic treatment is all the patient needs for a successful outcome.

Neck Pain and the Disk

When we say to you, "…you have a cervical disk problem," do you know what that means? I didn't think so. As doctors, we talk about these things so often, we sometimes just assume you know what we're talking about. So first, sorry about that! Now, let's clear up the question, what is a cervical disk problem?

The term "cervical" means neck, just like the terms "thoracic" means mid-back and "lumbar" means low back. The term "disk" refers to the shock absorbing fibro-elastic cartilage that rests between each vertebra of the spine. Think of the disk as being similar to a jelly donut. The center of the disk is liquid-like (the nucleus), kind of like petroleum jelly, and the outer part (the annulus) is tough and strong and circles the nucleus center like the rings of a freshly cut oak tree stump. What makes the annulus/outer layer so strong is the type of tissue it's made up of and, maybe most important, the opposing crisscross pattern of each layer or ring of the annulus. Studies have shown that when the disk is pierced with a knife and then compressed, this crisscross pattern of the annulus layers self-seals the cut, resulting in no leakage of the liquid center.

So, the question is, how can a disk rupture, herniate or "slip" if it's so tough, strong, and self-sealing? The answer: as the disk ages or when it's injured, tears or "fissures" in the disk fibers occur creating rents or channels for the liquid part to work its way out towards the edge and eventually break through the outer most layer – hence, the term "herniated disk." It's similar to stepping on that jelly

215

donut until the jelly leaks out to the point where you can see it.

Here's the strange part. Research tells us that about 50% of people have bulging disks (not quite herniated through) and 20% of us have herniated disks (that have popped through) but have NO PAIN AT ALL! That makes it tough since an MRI or CT scan may show a herniated or bulging disk but how do we know that's the disk that's clinically important – the one that's creating the pain? That's why we treat patients and not their image (MRI, CT scan or x-ray). Even though a disk may be bulging or herniated, we may not necessarily treat that particular disk if it's not expressing itself clinically by creating a shooting pain down a specific area in an arm, usually below the elbow often into either the thumb or pinky side of the hand, with associated abnormal tests for strength and/or sensation. That's why we check your reflexes, your strength, and sensation for each nerve. We're checking to see if that herniated disk is "pinching" the nerve and if it is, we utilize manipulation, traction, PT modalities, and issue home traction units to try to "un-pinch" that nerve to avoid surgery.

Neck Pain and Arthritis

When we say the word "arthritis," many images pop up in our heads. Some people think of crippled hands or perhaps Mr. Smith who talks about his bad hip being, "...bone on bone!" Or, how about the neighbor who has a bum knee and walks with a limp and a cane? Rarely do we think about the **neck** being associated with "arthritis."

Before we go too far into this discussion, we should define the term, "arthritis," which means joint ("arth-") swelling (-itis). Simple enough, right? Wrong! Without getting too complicated, we must realize there are MANY different types of arthritis such as osteoarthritis, rheumatoid arthritis, lupus, gouty arthritis, psoriatic arthritis, etc. To narrow this down a bit, we will limit our discussion to osteoarthritis, also known as degenerative joint disease.

Degenerative joint disease or DJD, is the most common type of arthritis that EVERYONE eventually ends up with – whether we like it or not. That's because, over time, our joints wear out and become "arthritic." While it's true that weight bearing joints wear out quicker (like hips and knees more so than elbows and shoulders), DJD can affect any joint. There are many causes of DJD, including a genetic or hereditary tendency but the most common cause is wear and tear over a long period of time. Of course, the rate of acquiring DJD in the neck (or anywhere else for that matter) is directly related to how "nice" we have been to our body, in this case, the neck. For example, after a car accident, a common injury to the neck is whiplash. This occurs because we literally cannot control the speed of the head as it rapidly moves forwards and backwards upon impact and it's all over within 600-800 milliseconds! Since we can't voluntarily contract a muscle that fast and when joints move beyond their normal stretch length, the ligaments – those non-elastic, tough tissues that securely holds bone to bone – will only "give" so much and then tear, which is technically called a "sprain." This leads to an accelerated rate of degeneration.

Blood tests are negative with DJD (unlike many of the other types of arthritis), and an x-ray can help determine how "arthritic" the joint is and whether the smooth, silky ends of the joint (called hyaline cartilage) are worn down and if bony spurs are present. In the neck, DJD can create a lot of symptoms which may include pain and stiffness, especially in the mornings after laying still and not moving during the night. After we get up and move around, "...it loosens up." As the condition advances, neck movements become tight and restricted with pain, which further limits movement, and sooner or later, the patient must rotate their whole body to look to the side. If the arthritis hits or bumps into a nerve as it exits the cervical spine, neck soreness, and numbness/tingling may radiate down an arm, at times to the hand, usually only affecting certain fingers. Headaches, especially in the back of the head, can also occur from the reflex muscle "splinting" due to the pain associated with arthritis. As Dr. Peter Ulrich, MD points out (http://www.spine-health.com/conditions/arthritis/cervical-osteoarthritis-neck-arthritis) chiropractic adjustments, "...help control chronic symptoms or provide relief for more severe episodes of pain from osteoarthritis."

Neck Pain: What Can I Do About It?

Neck pain is one of those conditions that affect most people at some point during their lifetime. All you have to do is ask just about anyone, "...have you ever had neck pain?" Then again, maybe you shouldn't since you'll probably get overloaded with way too much information from several people willing to share every little detail with you. Because of the way we are anatomically built, the neck is particularly vulnerable to injury (it has to hold up an average head weight of 15 pounds which can be quite a job, especially when we slump or slouch and that 15 pound weight falls forwards). Injury to the neck can result in minimal symptoms all the way to complete disability, making it one of the most common reasons people see doctors of all varieties for help. Couple neck pain with headaches and now you have a real potential for disrupting lifestyles. With simple causes like poor posture, stress, work station problems or long hours at a computer, not to mention anxiety, depression and more, it's no wonder most of us have needed help for neck pain at some point in time. So, the question remains, "…what can I do about it?"

From a chiropractic standpoint, manipulation, massage and other soft tissue techniques, and several forms of physiological therapeutics (such as ultrasound, electric stimulation, light – low level laser therapies), all work great! But, instead of (or, in addition to) things that WE do to you, let's discuss things we can teach YOU to do on your own. There is a long list of aids that help neck pain that you can self-manage, of which some include: a home traction device, cervical pillows, exercises, posture retraining, stress management, work station modifications, work / job analysis and subsequent modifications, and more. Most important is that YOU are in control of your own management program. All you need is a little motivation (your job) and proper training (our job). Many of these "self-help approaches" include an apparatus or device of some sort, which are technically coined, "hard durable medical supplies." More specifically: Cervical traction units include (but are not limited to) inflatable collars, seated over-the-door traction units, laying on the back varieties, as well as towel traction. The concept here is that you are stretching the neck vertebra apart and if it's done proper, it should feel good! Don't do it if it doesn't or, reduce the weight until it does feel good. Another type of traction is placing a fulcrum (dense foam triangle) behind the neck while lying allowing the head to hang off the edge of the bed.

1. Cervical pillows share the common concept of being contoured to fit the neck and head. These are thicker on the edge so the gap between the neck and shoulder point is filled in so the head is pointed straight ahead. There are many types of contoured pillows including water pillows, foam, inflatable, buckwheat, rice, and other types. However, a word of caution is in order: you may not like it at first as it can take 3-4 nights to get used to it. But, once you do, you'll miss your pillow when you're not able to travel with it.
2. Exercises. Place your hand against your head and push into the hand, allowing the head to "win" as you move through the full range of motion (forwards, backwards, sideways and rotation). Don't forget stretching, other strengthening exercises, and fine motor control exercises are important as well. We'll have to pick this topic up again in the near future.

"My Neck Is Killing Me!"

When patients present with **neck pain**, they always ask, "where is the pain coming from?" Of course, this can only be answered after a careful history and thorough evaluation is completed, which is what we do in this office. Let's take a closer look at what this involves.

The History : This includes a careful description of how the injury occurred, if there was an injury. For example, in a slip and fall injury, it makes a difference if the patient fell forwards, sideways, or backwards; if they landed on their knees, hips, buttocks, back or if they hit their head on the ground. Also, if there was a dazed feeling or loss of consciousness in the process. If there was a head strike, were there any signs of concussion: fatigue, mental "fog," headache, difficulty communicating or forming words or sentences. When there is no specific injury, we will ask if there were perhaps one or more, "mini-" or "micro-" injuries that may have occurred sometime within 2-3 days prior to the onset of the neck pain. The cumulative effect of several small "micro-injuries" can result in a rather significant onset of symptoms several days later. The next batch of information gathered includes factors that increase and decrease the pain, the type of pain quality (sharp, dull, throb, burn, itch, etc.), pain location – "...put your finger on where it hurts and "does it radiate into the arms or legs, severity (pain level 0-10), and timing such as, "it's worse for the 1st 30 min. in the morning and then loosens up." Information regarding past history, family history, medical history (surgeries, medications), social history, habits (caffeine, tobacco, alcohol, etc.), and a systems review (heart, lungs, stomach, nervous system, etc.).

The Physical Exam : This includes vital signs (blood pressure, etc.), observation – the way the head is positioned (forwards, to the side, rotated, etc.); palpation – touch/feel for muscle spasm, trigger points, spinal vertebra position and motion; range of motion, orthopedic and neurological tests. The exam procedure may also include x-ray, depending on each case.

The Diagnosis : This is determined after taking all your information and "...putting the puzzle pieces together" to determine what is causing your pain.

The Treatment : Chiropractic spinal manipulation (often referred to as "adjustments") is performed by applying energy or force to the misaligned or fixed vertebra structures by one of many methods depending on the patient's size, pain level, tolerance, and so on. Other "manual" treatment approaches include soft tissue therapy such as trigger point therapy, active release, massage, vibration, and others. The use of physical therapy modalities such as ice, heat, electrical stimulation, ultrasound, light – laser therapy, and/or others, again, depending on your specific situation and needs can also be very helpful. Similarly, exercises to teach you how to hold your proper posture, to improve flexibility or range of motion, and to strengthen the muscles that are weak really help to make the adjustments "hold" and the beneficial effects last longer. A work station/job assessment may also be needed if that appears to be irritating your condition.

Neck Pain Self-Help Techniques

It is very important that those of us with **neck pain** learn what we can do to help ourselves as the benefits from treatment are always much more satisfying for both the healthcare provider and patient. Self-care promotes independence and a feeling of accomplishment. You are the most important part of this "team" effort as we both work hard to "...get you better!" Let's take a look at what self-help techniques you can apply when neck pain strikes:

1. Acute stage : This is the period of time when neck pain first starts and it's usually very sore and painful. This stage occurs immediately after an injury and continues for 24 to 48 hours but can be perpetuated for a week or longer if you are careless about your activities and keep irritating it. Injuries to the neck are similar to a cut on the skin. If you pick your cut, it will bleed again. Sometimes, you have to wait a week or two before you can, "...pick off the scab." This analogy also applies to neck pain after an injury. At this stage, you need to apply the principle of "PRICE" (Protect, Rest, Ice, Compress, Elevate). OK, I guess we're not going to "compress" or "elevate" our neck but certainly the others apply nicely. To protect the neck, avoid quick/unguarded movements as these can "...pick at the cut" and re-injure the tissue. Rest means you may have to hold back on some activities that are strainful and might also, "....pick at the cut." Ice is a WONDERFUL pain killer and anti-inflammatory and should be rotated on/off/on/off/on at 15 minute rotations of ice/no ice/ice/no ice/ice. This creates a "pump-like" action that pushes away the swelling and therefore, reduces pain. After 24-48 hours, you can alternate ice/heat/ice/heat/ice at 10/5/10/5/10 minute intervals as heat relaxes tight muscles and as a result, can help reduce pain. These self-help techniques can continue for a few days to a whole month, depending on the degree of injury and, how "nice you are" to yourself (so you don't overdo it!) Cervical traction (home over-the-door traction) can really help a lot too!

2. Sub-acute stage : This stage of healing starts any time after 48-72 hours and can last 4-6 weeks or more, depending on again, the degree of injury and is "niceness" dependent! During this stage, the callus (scab) is hardening and its becoming stronger/less likely to "re-bleed." During this stage, range of motion, fiber stretching, isometric exercises can slowly be integrated into your program. Progressively harder exercises and re-introduction back into "normal" activities should be emphasized during this stage.
3. Chronic stage : This stage can last from 8 weeks to 1 or more years. When neck pain persists, determine which desired activities are well tolerated, including exercises. When "flare-ups" occur, a brief time period with PRI(CE) is nice! Exercises here can be quite physical and progressive, based on your tolerance and exercise experience.

Neck Pain Reducing Tricks

As stated last month, exercises that focus on improving posture, flexibility, strength, and coordination are important for creating a well-rounded cervical rehabilitation program. Our discussion continues this month with stretching and strengthening exercises.

STRETCHING: Since our neck muscles have to hold up our 12 pound (~5.5 kg) head, it's no wonder why our neck muscles seem to be tight almost all the time.

Here are two ways to stretch the neck:

1. You can simply drop the chin to the chest, look at the ceiling, try to touch your ear to your shoulder (without shoulder shrugging) on both sides, and rotate the head left to right and vice versa (six directions).
2. You can use gentle pressure with your hand and assist in the active stretch by gently pulling into the six directions described in #1 by applying "over-pressure" at the end-range of motion (staying within "reasonable pain boundaries").

STRENGTHENING: Most people have a forward head carriage, meaning their head normally rests in front of their shoulders. The further forward the head sits, the greater the load on the muscles in the back of the neck and upper back to hold it up. This position promotes a negative spiral or "vicious cycle" that can lead to many complaints including (but not limited to) neck pain, headaches, balance disturbances, and in the long-term, osteoarthritis.

There are two important groups of muscles that require strengthening: the deep neck flexors and deep neck extensors.

1. The deep neck flexors are muscles located directly on the front of the cervical spine and are described as being "involuntary" or unable to be voluntarily contracted. Hence, we have to "trick" the voluntary outer "extrinsic" (stronger) muscles into NOT WORKING so the deep, intrinsic ones will contract. You can do this by flexing your chin to the chest and pushing your neck (not head) back over your shoulders into resistance caused a towel wrapped around the back of the neck. If you feel your chin rise towards the ceiling, you're doing it WRONG!

225

Keep the chin tucked as close to the chest as possible as you push your neck (not your head) backwards. If you're doing it correctly, your chest should rise towards the ceiling as you push your chin down and neck back. Try it!

2. The deep neck extensors are strengthened in a very similar way EXCEPT here you DO push the back of HEAD back into your towel while keeping your chin tucked tightly into your chest. Do three reps, holding each for three to five seconds and switch between the two for two to three sets.

Neck Pain – Management Strategies

As discussed last month, when you make an appointment for a chiropractic evaluation for your neck pain, your doctor of chiropractic will provide both in-office procedures as well as teach you many self-help approaches so that as a "team", together WE can manage your neck pain or headache complaint to a satisfying end-point. So, what are some of these procedures? Let's take a look!

In the office, you can expect to receive a thorough history, examination, x-ray (if warranted), and a discussion about what chiropractic care can be done for you and your condition. Your doctor will map out a treatment plan and discuss commonly shared goals of 1) Pain reduction, 2) Posture/alignment restoration, and 3) Prevention of future episodes. Pain reduction approaches include (but are not limited to) joint mobilization and/or manipulation, muscle/ligament stretching techniques, inflammation control by the use of physical therapy modalities (such as electrical stimulation), ice, and possibly anti-inflammatory vitamin / herbal therapies. Your chiropractor will also teach you proper body mechanics for bending/lifting/pulling/pushing, and help you avoid positions or situations where you might re-injure the area. Posture/alignment restoration can include methods such as spinal manipulation / mobilization and leg length correction strategies (heel and/or sole lifts, special orthotic shoes, and/or foot orthotic inserts). These are often GREAT recommendations as they "work" all the time they are in your shoes and you don't have to do anything (except wear them)! The third goal of future episode prevention is often a combination ongoing treatment in the office and strategies you can employ at home. This includes (but is not limited to): 1) whether you should use ice, heat, or both at times of acute exacerbation; 2) avoiding positions or movements that create sharp/lancinating pain; 3) DOING THE EXERCISES that you've been taught ON A REGULAR BASIS; and 4) eating and an "anti-inflammatory" diet (lean meats, lots of fruits/veggies, and avoid gluten – wheat, oats, barley, rye).

Let's talk exercise! Your doctor of chiropractic will teach you exercises that are designed to increase range of motion (ROM), re-educate a flat or reversed curve in the neck, and strengthen / stabilize the muscles in the neck. Studies show that the deep neck flexor muscles – those that are located deep, next to the spine in the front of the neck – are frequently weak in patients with neck pain. These muscles are NOT voluntary so you have to "trick" them into contracting with very specific exercises. Your doctor will also teach you exercises that you can do EVERY HOUR of your work day (for 10-15 seconds) that are designed to prevent neck pain from gradually worsening so you aren't miserable by the end of work. Along these lines, he/she will discuss the set-up of your work station and how you might improve it – whether it's a chair, desk, computer position, a table/work station height issue, or a reaching problem; using proper "ergonomics" can REALLY HELP! Your doctor will also advise you not to talk on the phone pinching the receiver between your head and shoulder, to face the person you are talking to (avoiding prolonged head rotation), to tuck in your chin as a posture training exercise, and more. Cervical traction can be a GREAT home-applied, self-help strategy, and these come in many varieties. Proper positions for the head when sleeping and a properly fitted contoured pillow is also important since we spend about 1/3 of our lives asleep!

Neck Pain Reducing "Tricks" (Part 3 of 3)

This series has included exercise recommendations to self-manage neck pain, headache, upper back pain, and dizziness. This month's topic involves enhancing coordination, which may be the most important topic in this three-part series!

Coordination-based exercises are important because they stimulate our neuro-motor system and can help restore normal function. We can all relate to the challenge of learning new activities. In many cases, we may struggle with the basics, but over time, they become easier to perform and we're eventually able to accomplish these neuromuscular sequences without even thinking about it.

When we are injured, we COMPENSATE and change our methods of doing the various tasks associated with our work and daily living. Unfortunately, these altered neuromotor sequences can become our "new normal" and can lead to other faulty compensatory motor functions (a negative vicious cycle). To "fix" this, we must First "Identify" the faulty pattern, Second "Fix" the faulty pattern consciously, Third "Practice" the new or proper method long enough so that, Fourth The proper/new/fixed method becomes automatic or "unconscious." So, HOW do we re-establish proper motor function after an injury?

We can all start stimulating the neuromotor system by adding coordination-based components to our current fitness program. For example, when performing an exercise, release slowly but keep resisting. This "eccentric" resistance (resistance as the muscle elongates) builds coordination while the "concentric" resistance (resistance as the muscle shortens/contracts) builds strength. Apply this principle to ALL resistance exercises, and remember only use a light amount of resistance when exercising your neck muscles – only 10-20% of a maximum push! Another "principle" that is applicable to ALL exercises is to start simple and slowly add or integrate more complex movements or start doing two things at once (like pinch a ball between your knees or stand on one leg while performing your neck exercises). Be "mindful" or THINK about what you are doing to further stimulate the nervous system. Some other ways to add variety to your exercises include incorporating sitting on a gym ball, jumping, or standing on a rocker or wobble board. MAKE IT FUN and challenging! ALWAYS build on what you have previously mastered!

Exercises for Improving Cervical Posture

Is there a "normal" or "best posture" out there? If so, what is it?

Posture is largely inherited; however, there are also environmental, social, and other forces that can affect posture. Some say "good posture" is the position that places the least amount of strain on the body, particularly the muscles and ligaments that hold the body together.

A common cause of poor posture is called forward head carriage (FHC), where the head sits forward of the shoulders, placing a greater strain on the back of the neck and upper back to hold the head upright. Looking at the spine from the side, the opening of the ear should line up with the shoulder, hip, and ankle.

There have been studies that suggest every inch (2.54 cm) of FHC increases muscle strain in neck and upper back by 10 pounds (4.5 kg). That means a 5 inch (~12.7 cm) FHC adds an extra 50 pounds (~22.7 kg) of strain on the neck and upper back to hold the head upright. So what can we do to improve our posture?

First, stay active to reduce the normal rate of degeneration that affects us all as we "mature" through life! This recommendation requires us to keep fit and strive to maintain a normal BMI ("body mass index" or weight/height ratio) by balancing calorie intake and exercise.

Now, besides being evaluated for specific spinal care, there are a couple exercises you can do to help improve your cervical posture:

EXERCISE #1 is called a chin tuck. Here, you simply pull your chin inwards, producing a "double chin." If you do this as far as you can and talk your voice will sound funny ("nasal-like"). Release the tuck until your voice clears. The moment it clears, STOP – that's your "new" head position. Try to maintain that all day. You will have to remind yourself to "…keep it tucked" frequently at first but as time goes on, it will feel more natural. This can take about three months on average, so BE PATIENT!

EXERCISE #2 will strengthen the deep neck flexor muscles by doing the exact same thing as exercise #1 BUT adds a hand, a towel, or a TheraBand (anything works) for resistance behind the neck so that as you chin tuck, you PRESS the back of your mid-neck into your finger tips (or Band, towel, etc.) and hold for five seconds (then, release slowly). Do this five, ten, or multiple times a day.

There are other exercises but this is a GREAT start! See your doctor of chiropractic for more specific individual needs!

REFERENCES

Kirkaldy-Willis WH, Cassidy, JD; Spinal Manipulation in the Treatment of Low back Pain; Canadian Family Physician; March 1985, Vol. 31, pp. 535-540.

Ramsey RH; Conservative Treatment of Intervertebral Disk Lesions; American Academy of Orthopedic Surgeons, Instructional Course Lectures; Volume 11, 1954, pp. 118-120.

Mathews JA and Yates DAH; Reduction of Lumbar Disc Prolapse by Manipulation; British Medical Journal; September 20, 1969, No. 3, 696-697.

Edwards BC; Low back pain and pain resulting from lumbar spine conditions: a comparison of treatment results; Australian Journal of Physiotherapy; 15:104, 1969.

White AA, Panjabi MM; Clinical Biomechanics of the Spine ; Second edition, JB Lippincott Company, 1990.

Turek S; Orthopedics, Principles and Their Applications ; JB Lippincott Company; 1977; page 1335.

Kuo PP and Loh ZC; Treatment of Lumbar Intervertebral Disc Protrusions by Manipulation; Clinical Orthopedics and Related Research. No. 215, February 1987, pp. 47-55.

Quon JA, Cassidy JD, O'Connor SM, Kirkaldy-Willis WH; Lumbar intervertebral disc herniation: treatment by rotational manipulation; Journal of Manipulative and Physiological Therapeutics; 1989 Jun;12(3):220-7.

Cassidy JD, Thiel HW, Kirkaldy-Willis WH; Side posture manipulation for lumbar intervertebral disk herniation; Journal of Manipulative and Physiological Therapeutics; February 1993;16(2):96-103.

Stern PJ, Côté P, Cassidy JD; A series of consecutive cases of low back pain with radiating leg pain treated by chiropractors; Journal of Manipulative and Physiological Therapeutics; 1995 Jul-Aug;18(6):335-42.

Santilli V, Beghi E, Finucci S; Chiropractic manipulation in the treatment of acute back pain and sciatica with disc protrusion: A randomized double-blind clinical trial of active and simulated spinal manipulations; The Spine Journal; March-April 2006; Vol. 6; No. 2; pp. 131–137.

Bronfort G, Hondras M, Schulz CA, Evans RL, Long CR, PhD; Grimm R; Spinal Manipulation and Home Exercise With Advice for Subacute and Chronic Back-Related Leg Pain; A Trial With Adaptive Allocation; Annals of Internal Medicine; September 16, 2014; Vol. 161; No. 6; pp. 381-391.

Leemann S, Peterson CK, Schmid C, Anklin B, Humphreys BK; Outcomes of Acute and Chronic Patients with Magnetic Resonance Imaging–Confirmed Symptomatic Lumbar Disc Herniations Receiving High-Velocity, Low Amplitude, Spinal Manipulative Therapy: A Prospective Observational Cohort Study With One-Year Follow-Up; Journal of Manipulative and Physiological Therapeutics; March/April 2014; Vol. 37; No. 3; pp. 155-163.

"Authored by Dan Murphy, D.C.. Published by ChiroTrust® – This publication is not meant to offer treatment advice or protocols. Cited material is not necessarily the opinion of the author or publisher."

1) Mixter WJ, Barr JS. Rupture of the Intervertebral Disc with Involvement of the Spinal Canal. New England Journal of Medicine. CCXI, 210, 1934.

2) Barr JS, Mixter WJ. Posterior Protrusion of the Lumbar Intervertebral Discs. Journal of Bone and Joint Surgery (American). 1941;23:444-456.

3) Nachemson AL, The Lumbar Spine: An Orthopedic Challenge. Spine, Volume 1, Number 1, March 1976, pp. 59-71.

4) Smyth MJ, Wright V, Sciatica and the intervertebral disc. An experimental study. Journal of Bone and Joint Surgery [American];40: 1958, pp. 1401-1408.

5) Bogduk N, Tynan W, Wilson AS. The nerve supply to the human lumbar intervertebral discs, Journal of Anatomy; 1981, 132, 1, pp. 39-56.

6) Bogduk N. The innervation of the lumbar spine. Spine. April 1983;8(3): pp. 286-93.

7) Mooney, V, Where Is the Pain Coming From? Spine, 12(8), 1987, pp. 754-759.

8) Kuslich S, Ulstrom C, Michael C; The Tissue Origin of Low Back Pain and Sciatica: A Report of Pain Response to Tissue Stimulation During Operations on the Lumbar Spine Using Local Anesthesia; Orthopedic Clinics of North America, Vol. 22, No. 2, April 1991, pp.181-7.

9) Ozawa, Tomoyuki MD; Ohtori, Seiji MD; Inoue, Gen MD; Aoki, Yasuchika MD; Moriya, Hideshige MD; Takahashi, Kazuhisa MD; The Degenerated Lumbar Intervertebral Disc is Innervated Primarily by Peptide-Containing Sensory Nerve Fibers in Humans; Spine, Volume 31(21), October 1, 2006, pp. 2418-2422.

10) Bogduk N, Aprill C. On the nature of neck pain, discography and cervical zygapophysial joint blocks; Pain; August 1993;54(2):213-7.

11) **Barnsley L, Lord SM, Wallis BJ, Bogduk N.** The prevalence of chronic cervical zygapophysial joint pain after whiplash. Spine. 1995 Jan 1;20(1):20-5.

12) **Lord SM, Barnsley L, Wallis BJ, Bogduk N**. Chronic cervical zygapophysial joint pain after whiplash. A placebo-controlled prevalence study. Spine. 1996 Aug 1;21(15):1737-44.

13) Indahl A, Kaigle A, Reikerås O, Holm S. **Electromyographic response of the porcine multifidus musculature after nerve stimulation.** Spine. 1995 Dec 15;20(24):2652-8.

14) Indahl A, Kaigle AM, Reikeras O et al (1997) Interaction between the porcine lumbar intervertebral disc, zygapophysial joints, and paraspinal muscles. Spine 22:2834–2840.

15) **The ligamento-muscular stabilizing system of the spine.** Solomonow M, Zhou BH, Harris M, Lu Y, Baratta RV. Spine. 1998 Dec 1;23(23):2552-62.

16) Panjabi MM. **A hypothesis of chronic back pain: ligament subfailure injuries lead to muscle control dysfunction.** Eur Spine J. 2006 May;15(5):668-76.

17) Barnsley L, Lord SM, Wallis BJ, Bogduk N. **Lack of effect of intraarticular corticosteroids for chronic pain in the cervical zygapophyseal joints.** N Engl J Med. 1994 Apr 14;330(15):1047-50.

18) Kirkaldy-Willis, W.H., M.D., & Cassidy, J.D.,"Spinal Manipulation in the Treatment of Low-Back Pain," Can Fam Physician, (1985), 31:535-40.

19) Hoving JL, Koes BW, de Vet HCW, van der Windt AWM, Assendelft WJJ, van Mameren H, Devillé WLJM, Pool JJM, Scholten RJPM,Bouter LM. Manual Therapy, Physical Therapy, or Continued Care by a General Practitioner for Patients with Neck Pain A Randomized, Controlled Trial. Annals of Internal Medicine, Vol. 136 No. 10, Pages 713-722 May 21, 2002.

1) Mixter WJ, Barr JS; Rupture of the intervertebral disc with involvement of the spinal canal; New England Journal of Medicine; 211 (1934), pp. 210–215.

2) Inman VT, and Saunders JMB, Anatamico-physiological aspects of injuries to the inververtebral disc, J Bone Joint Surg 29 (1947), pp. 461–468.

3) Nachemson, AL, Spine, Volume 1, Number 1, March 1976, pp. 59-71.

4) Smyth MJ, Wright V, Sciatica and the intervertebral disc. An experimental study. Journal of Bone and Joint Surgery [American]; Vol. 40, No. 6. December 1958, pp. 1401-1418.

5) Jayson M, Editor; The Lumbar Spine and Back Pain , Third Edition, Churchill Livingstone, 1987, p. 60.

6) Bogduk N, Tynan W, Wilson AS, The nerve supply to the human lumbar intervertebral discs, Journal of Anatomy; 1981, 132, 1, pp. 39-56.

7) Bogduk N, The innervation of the lumbar spine; Spine. April 1983;8(3): pp. 286-93.

8) Mooney, V, Where Is the Pain Coming From? Spine, 12(8), 1987, pp. 754-759.

9) Kuslich S, Ulstrom C, Michael C; The Tissue Origin of Low Back Pain and Sciatica: A Report of Pain Response to Tissue Stimulation During Operations on the Lumbar Spine Using Local Anesthesia; Orthopedic Clinics of North America, Vol. 22, No. 2, April 1991, pp.181-7,

10) Ozawa, Tomoyuki MD; Ohtori, Seiji MD; Inoue, Gen MD; Aoki, Yasuchika MD; Moriya, Hideshige MD; Takahashi, Kazuhisa MD; The Degenerated Lumbar Intervertebral Disc is Innervated Primarily by Peptide-Containing Sensory Nerve Fibers in Humans; Spine, Volume 31(21), October 1, 2006, pp. 2418-2422.

11) Kirkaldy-Willis WH, Cassidy JD; Spinal Manipulation in the Treatment of Low Back Pain; Canadian Family Physician, March 1985, Vol. 31, pp. 535-540

12) Meade TW, Dyer S, Browne W, Townsend J, Frank OA; Low back pain of mechanical origin: Randomized comparison of chiropractic and hospital outpatient treatment; British Medical Journal; Volume 300, June 2, 1990, pp. 1431-7.

13) Giles LGF, Muller R; Chronic Spinal Pain: A Randomized Clinical Trial Comparing Medication, Acupuncture, and Spinal Manipulation; Spine, July 15, 2003; 28(14):1490-1502.

14) Muller R, Lynton G.F. Giles LGF, DC, PhD; Long-Term Follow-up of a Randomized Clinical Trial Assessing the Efficacy of Medication, Acupuncture, and Spinal Manipulation for Chronic Mechanical Spinal Pain Syndromes; Journal of Manipulative and Physiological Therapeutics, January 2005, Volume 28, No. 1.

15) Roger Chou, MD; Amir Qaseem, MD, PhD, MHA; Vincenza Snow, MD; Donald Casey, MD, MPH, MBA; J. Thomas Cross Jr., MD, MPH; Paul Shekelle,

235

MD, PhD; and Douglas K. Owens, MD, MS; Diagnosis and Treatment of Low Back Pain; Annals of Internal Medicine; Volume 147, Number 7, October 2007, pp. 478-491.

16) Roger Chou, MD, and Laurie Hoyt Huffman, MS; Nonpharmacologic Therapies for Acute and Chronic Low Back Pain; Annals of Internal Medicine; October 2007, Volume 147, Number 7, pp. 492-504.

17) Kirkaldy-Willis WH, Managing Low Back Pain , Churchill Livingstone, 1983, p. 19.

18) Gargan MF, Bannister GC; Long-Term Prognosis of Soft-Tissue Injuries of the Neck; Journal of Bone and Joint Surgery (British); Vol. 72-B, No. 5, September 1990, pp. 901-3.

19) Chance GQ; Note on a type of flexion fracture of the spine; British Journal of Radiology; September 1948, No. 21, pp. 452-453.

20) Howland WJ, Curry JL, Buffington CB. Fulcrum fractures of the lumbar spine. JAMA. 1965 Jul 19;193:240-1.

21) Rennie W, Mitchell N. **Flexion distraction fractures of the thoracolumbar spine.** J Bone Joint Surg Am. 1973 Mar;55(2):386-90.

22) Murphy DJ; "Children in Motor Vehicle Collisions", in Pediatric Chiropractic , Edited by Anrig C and Plaugher G; Williams & Wilkins, 1998.

1) Foreman J; Why Women are Living in the Discomfort Zone; More Than 100 Million American Adults Live with Chronic Pain—Most of them Women. What will it take to bring them relief?; January 31, 2014.

2) Wang S; Why Does Chronic Pain Hurt Some People More?; Wall Street Journal; October 7, 2013.

3) Pho, K; USA TODAY, The Forum; September 19, 2011; pg. 9A.

4) Nachemson, Alf, MD, PhD; The Lumbar Spine, An Orthopedic Challenge; SPINE Volume 1, Number 1, March 1976, Pages 59-71.

5) White AA, Panjabi MM, Clinical Biomechanics of the Spine , Second Edition, J.B. Lippincott Company, 1990.

6) Croft PR, Macfarlane GJ, Papageorgiou AC, Thomas E, Silman AJ; Outcome of Low Back Pain in General Practice: A Prospective Study; British Medical Journal; May 2, 1998; Vol. 316, pp. 1356-

7) Hestbaek L, Leboeuf-Yde C, Manniche C; Low back pain: what is the long-term course? A review of studies of general patient populations; European Spine Journal; April 2003; Vol. 12; No 2; pp. 149-65.

8) Donelson R, McIntosh G; Hall H; Is It Time to Rethink the Typical Course of Low Back Pain?; Physical Medicine and Rehabilitation (PM&R); Vol. 4; No. 6; June 2012, Pages 394–401.

9) Itz CJ, Geurts JW, van Kleef M, Nelemans P; Clinical course of non-specific low back pain: a systematic review of prospective cohort studies set in primary care; European Journal of Pain; January 2013;Vol. 17; No. 1; pp. 5-15.

10) Dunn KM, Hestbaek L, Cassidy JD; Low back pain across the life course;Best Practice & Research Clinical Rheumatology; October 2013; Vol. 27; No. 5; pp. 591-600.

11) Cifuentes M, Willetts J, Wasiak R; Health Maintenance Care in Work-Related Low Back Pain and Its Association With Disability Recurrence; Journal of Occupational and Environmental Medicine; April 14, 2011; Vol. 53; No. 4; pp. 396-404.

12) Senna MK, Machaly SA; Does Maintained Spinal Manipulation Therapy for Chronic Nonspecific Low Back Pain Result in Better Long-Term Outcome? Randomized Trial; SPINE; August 15, 2011; Volume 36, Number 18, pp. 1427–1437.

1) Cyriax, James; Textbook of Orthopedic Medicine, Diagnosis of Soft Tissue Lesions , Bailliere Tindall, Volume 1, eighth edition, 1982.

2) Boyd, William, Pathology , Lea and Febiger, 1952.

3) Guyton, Arthur, Textbook of Medical Physiology , Saunders, 1986.

4) Roy, Steven; Irvin, Richard; Sports Medicine: Prevention, Evaluation, Management, and   Rehabilitation , Prentice-Hall, 1983.

5) Cohen, I. Kelman; Diegelmann, Robert F; Lindbald, William J; Wound Healing, Biochemical &   Clinical Aspects , WB Saunders, 1992.

6) Melham TJ, Sevier TL, Malnofski MJ, Wilson JK, Helfst RK, Chronic ankle pain and fibrosis successfully treated with a new noninvasive augmented soft tissue

mobilization technique (ASTM); Medicine Science Sports Exercise, June 1998; 30(3): 801-4.

7) Seletz E, Whiplash Injuries, Neurophysiological Basis for Pain and Methods Used for Rehabilitation; Journal of the American Medical Association, November 29, 1958, pp. 1750– 1755.

8) Stearns, ML, Studies on development of connective tissue in transparent chambers in rabbit's ear; American Journal of Anatomy, vol. 67, 1940, p. 55.

9) Kellett J, Acute soft tissue injuries–a review of the literature;

Medicine and Science in Sports and Exercise. Oct. 1986;18(5):489-500.

10) Jonsson H, Cesarini K, Sahlstedt B, Rauschning W, Findings and Outcome in Whiplash-Type Neck Distortions; Spine, Vol. 19, No. 24, December 15, 1994, pp 2733-2743.

11) Buckwalter J, Effects of Early Motion on Healing of Musculoskeletal Tissues, Hand Clinics, Volume 12, Number 1, February 1996.

12) Salter R, Continuous Passive Motion, A Biological Concept for the Healing and Regeneration of Articular Cartilage, Ligaments, and Tendons; From Origination to Research to Clinical Applications , Williams and Wilkins, 1993.

13) Kannus P, Immobilization or Early Mobilization After an Acute Soft-Tissue Injury?; The Physician And Sports Medicine; March, 2000; Vol. 26 No 3, pp. 55-63.

14) Mealy K, Brennan H, Fenelon GCC; Early Mobilization of Acute Whiplash Injuries; British Medical Journal, March 8, 1986, 292(6521): 656-657.

15) Rosenfeld M, Gunnarsson R, Borenstein P, Early Intervention in Whiplash-Associated Disorders, A Comparison of Two Treatment Protocols; Spine, 2000;25:1782-1787.

1) Nachemson, AL, Spine, Volume 1, Number 1, March 1976, pp. 59-71.

2) Smyth MJ, Wright V, Sciatica and the intervertebral disc. An experimental study. Journal of Bone and Joint Surgery [American];40: 1548, pp. 1401-1408.

3) Jayson M, Editor; The Lumbar Spine and back Pain, Third Edition, Churchill Livingstone, 1987, p. 60.

4) Bogduk N, Tynan W, Wilson A. S., The nerve supply to the human lumbar intervertebral discs, Journal of Anatomy. (1981, 132, 1, pp. 39-56.

238

5) Bogduk N., The innervation of the lumbar spine. Spine. April 1983;8(3): pp. 286-93.

6) Mooney, V, Where Is the Pain Coming From? Spine, 12(8), 1987, pp. 754-759.

7) Kuslich S, Ulstrom C, Michael C; The Tissue Origin of Low Back Pain and Sciatica: A Report of Pain Response to Tissue Stimulation During Operations on the Lumbar Spine Using Local Anesthesia;

8) Ozawa, Tomoyuki MD; Ohtori, Seiji MD; Inoue, Gen MD; Aoki, Yasuchika MD; Moriya, Hideshige MD; Takahashi, Kazuhisa MD; The Degenerated Lumbar Intervertebral Disc is Innervated Primarily by Peptide-Containing Sensory Nerve Fibers in Humans; Spine, Volume 31(21), October 1, 2006, pp. 2418-2422.

9) Kirkaldy-Willis WH, Cassidy JD; Spinal Manipulation in the Treatment of Low Back Pain; Canadian Family Physician, March 1985, Vol. 31, pp. 535-540

10) Meade TW, Dyer S, Browne W, Townsend J, Frank OA; Low back pain of mechanical origin: Randomized comparison of chiropractic and hospital outpatient treatment; British Medical Journal; Volume 300, June 2, 1990, pp. 1431-7.

11) Giles LGF, Muller R; Chronic Spinal Pain: A Randomized Clinical Trial Comparing Medication, 12) Muller R, Lynton G.F. Giles LGF, DC, PhD; Long-Term Follow-up of a Randomized Clinical Trial Assessing the Efficacy of Medication, Acupuncture, and Spinal Manipulation for Chronic Mechanical Spinal Pain Syndromes; Journal of Manipulative and Physiological Therapeutics, January 2005, Volume 28, No. 1.

13) Kirkaldy-Willis WH, Managing Low Back Pain , Churchill Livingstone, 1983, p.19.

See What Our Patients Have To Say...

"Dr. David Warwick took the time to learn about my injury and recommend my options. I started with a back adjustment, and it just felt a little better immediately afterwards. I woke up the next morning and felt way better. I am now convinced I will continue my treatment until I feel completely healed. Glad I went here and met with Dr. Warwick."

"I came, hesitantly, to Dr. Warwick's office due to pain, numbness, and tingling down both arms and limited range of motion in my neck and shoulders. I was not familiar with chiropractic as a medical option, but was faced with an ongoing treatment regimen of shots in my neck and limiting my activities, possibly forever. I decided I was not ready for that and needed a more logical, natural way to return to health. Needless to say, there has been great improvement not only in my neck and shoulders, but also lower back – discomfort I had just gotten used to. Dr. Warwick's willingness to really listen and understand my interest in a natural solution to regaining my health and strength has been empowering. Dr. Warwick is a medical provider, teacher, and true healer. THANK YOU!!!

"After my auto accident I experienced frequent and mysterious headaches. But not so mysterious for Dr. Warwick. He was knowledgeable, kind, and thoughtful in explaining to me my situation. Since seeing him, my headaches are gone. I feel confident in the care Dr. Warwick skillfully provides."

"Dr. David Warwick took the time to learn about my injury and recommend my options. I started with a back adjustment, and it just felt a little better immediately afterwards. I woke up the next morning and felt way better. I am now convinced I will continue my treatment until I feel completely healed. Glad I went here and met with Dr. Warwick."

"WOW! I am pain-free for the first time in two weeks! Thanks so much to Dr. David Warwick for an amazing job. I have so far to go, but now I am on the right track. I have been telling people for years that proper setup of a guitar is crucial to it playing well, just as a front alignment and tune up is to a car. It will work without it, but nowhere near its potential. All this time, my spine has been a disaster. The first visit, I knew I was on the right track. Treated like a welcomed guest, not as a number, and walking away with less pain and increased mobility. I had forgotten it was possible! Thank you so much!"

"I went into to meet with Dr. Warwick today, having been worked on by several massage therapists and Chiropractors over the years. I had a long relationship with my chiropractor and was really just trying something new and networking (I am a massage therapist) BUT Oh MY! He adjusted me today, found things I didn't realize were going on, relieved pain I wasn't really fully aware of and changed my entire day by lifting my mood and making my stress tolerable. I ended up with a smile for several hours just because I felt AMAZING! I will be singing his praises from the mountain top, As for my other chiro, well thanks for the memories but I am now a client of Dr. Warwick! If he can do that on my first visit, I can't wait to see what regular visits will do!"

"I don't do these often, so those who know me also know how much weight this carries. Highlight of my day today was probably the most no-nonsense, hassle-free, and delightful visit to the offices of my friend Dr. David Warwick to get a checkup of my lower back pain. No lectures, no suggestions of 20 "preventive" visits, just an honest diagnosis, some great pointers, a quick and effective adjustment, and out the door I went. For anyone seeking a fantastic chiropractor, please give Dr. Warwick a call; more than a Doc, the man is a breath of fresh air!"

"Dr. David is a miracle worker!! I saw him after having no idea how I injured my back and had seen another chiropractor twice..... but within two visits Dr. David had me walking, sitting, and sleeping pain free. Thank you Dr. David...you are simply the best!!"
"I have been in pain for a very long time but I went Dr. Warwick, and he was the only one that has helped me with my lower back pain. I will continue to keep on seeing him for as long as I can. Thank you, Dr. Warwick!"

"I have never felt better in years, I have suffered from neck pain for a long time. I have had numerous doctor visits and have always still had pain. I have been seeing Dr. Warwick and was pleasantly surprised of the relief I continue to have. I love, love, love the results!"

"I came in to see Dr. Warwick because I was suffering from Bell's Palsy. Almost immediately I started seeing results. I have now been going to Dr. Warwick for 2 ½ months, and I'm 100% back. I contribute that completely to the chiropractic work I have been doing. Not only that but I found out my body was lopsided, and I feel so much better. I haven't felt this good in ten years!"

"Dr. Warwick is very kind, attentive and professional. He always asks how I am feeling and if the chiropractic work he offers is helpful to me and my health. I really appreciate his professionalism, care and knowledge. I would happily refer him to all my friends!"

"Dr. Warwick is so dedicated to your health and happiness. It has been a pleasure being treated by him and others on the staff.

I have suffered from back pain for several years. I have seen multiple chiropractors, doctors, massage therapists, and acupuncturists. I even had 3 back injections! All provided no relief. I saw Dr. Warwick ONE time and I was pain free for 12 hours, which was the first time I had been pain free in years! After 3 treatments I was pain free for a week! HIGHLY RECOMMEND!!

Today was my first time ever going into a chiropractic office, I was so nervous at first, but when Dr. David M Warwick talked to me about what was going to be done I was comfortable. He was very quick and gentle and the relief of 9 years of tension, misalignment, and stress in my neck, mid, and lower back was instantly gone. I would recommend him to anyone to go to. I seriously feel so much better for the first time in a long time thanks to him!

1st time ever to see a chiropractor & Dr. Warwick has done an amazing job with adjusting my lower back! He has been very explanatory & most of all patient with me as I learn the process for what needs to be done. I really like the option of either walking in or making an appt. online too!

I have been seeing Dr. Warwick for 9 months now. I work in a physically demanding job with a lot of repetitive motion that has taken a toll on my body. Dr. Warwick has provided me with exceptional treatment and it truly is a joy to see him knowing that I have been given back my freedom of movement and my pain is now under control. I highly recommend Dr Warwick to anyone seeking excellent chiropractic care

I felt 2 inches taller. Finally someone noticed my poor posture and recognized the pain that was there!

Dr. Warwick has been a godsend. I still play competitive baseball in my late 30's, and deal with a painful back injury, but after a visit to his office, I can not only walk out under my own power, but am ready to compete at the level I've been accustomed to my whole life. So very glad that he is here.

I was so scared to see a Chiropractor, but Dr. Warwick made my first visit very comfortable, explaining everything step by step! Now that I have gone to him a few times, I really feel like the ease of scheduling online and how AMAZING I feel after every visit is well worth the small amount of money I pay to feel great!

I feel very fortunate to have found Warwick Chiropractic. I've been to several chiropractors over the years, but Dr. Warwick's technique and bedside manner are unlike any other. He addresses all of my concerns, he listens to my needs and makes sure that I'm comfortable! I entrust him with my children's Chiropractic needs as well!

Dr. Warwick is genuine and honest. He spent time really evaluating my pain and adjusting specific to what I needed, not just the normal 3 chiropractor adjustments.

I haven't been able to lift my right arm straight up for almost a decade... after just one visit, I can reach straight up!! I'm so thankful to have found Dr. Warwick and will be back again next week for a follow up. Thank you so much!

I am grateful to Dr. Warwick for the knowledge he gave me and for his care and thoroughness in administering my alignment . This was my first visit. WOW ! WONDERFUL ! RESTORATIVE !

Dr. David Warwick at Warwick Chiropractic

Your Local Lacey / Olympia WA Chiropractor
Short Term Care for Your Back & Neck Pain
Thurston County Auto Accident Pain Relief Specialist

Walk-Ins Welcome - No Appointment Needed
Simple & Convenient On-Line Scheduling

Visit my website www.DrDavidWarwick.com
Office: 8650 Martin Way East #207, Lacey WA 98516
Call 360-951-4504

Like Us on Facebook: **Warwick Chiropractic PLLC**

Watch my YouTube Videos for Great Tips and Live Treatments on **Warwick Chiropractic – Dr David Warwick Lacey Chiropractor**

For More Great Articles, Visit my Blog Page
www.DrDavidWarwick.com & www.DrDavidWarwickBlog.com

Grab My FREE Relief Books
Back & Neck Pain Relief
http://backandneckpainrelieflaceychiropractor.com/
You're Not A Dummy..Washington's Health Guide For Car Accident Victims
http://yourenotadummywahealthguideforcaraccidentvictims.com/

You Can Also Sign Up for my Pain Relief Email Updates & Monthly Newsletter at www.DrDavidWarwick.com

Thank you for Subscribing to my YouTube Channel, Facebook Page, Pain Relief Updates, and Monthly Newsletter. Thank you for taking your time to comment and enjoy.....See You Soon!

Questions for Dr. Warwick:

Made in the USA
Monee, IL
22 February 2020